Atlas of Coronary Artery Disease

Atlas of Coronary Artery Disease

Michael J. Davies, M.D., F.R.C.P., F.A.C.C., **F.E.C.C., F.R.C. Path.**

Professor
British Heart Foundation Cardiovascular Pathology Unit
St. George's Hospital Medical School
London, United Kingdom

with a contribution by
Siew Yen Ho, Ph.D., F.R.C. Path.

Senior Lecturer
Department of Pediatric Cardiac Morphology
Imperial College School of Medicine
National Heart and Lung Institute
London, United Kingdom

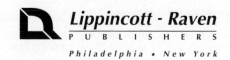

Lippincott - Raven
P U B L I S H E R S
Philadelphia • New York

Acquisitions Editor: Ruth W. Weinberg
Developmental Editor: Anne Snyder
Manufacturing Manager: Dennis Teston
Production Manager: Jodi Borgenicht
Production Editor: Deirdre Marino-Vasquez
Cover Designer: Karen Quigley
Indexer: Frances Lennie
Compositor: Lippincott–Raven Desktop Division

Printed and bound in China

9 8 7 6 5 4 3 2 1

Library of Congress Cataloging-in-Publication Data

Davies, M. J.
    Atlas of coronary artery disease / M. J. Davies : with a contribution by Siew Yen Ho.
        p.   c.m.
    Includes index.
    ISBN 0-397-58750-3
    1. Coronary heart disease—Atlases.   I. Ho, Siew Yen.   II. Title.
    [DNLM: 1. Coronary Disease—pathology atlases.
    2. Atherosclerosis—pathology atlases.   WG 17 D256a 1998]
RC685.C6D385   1998
616.1'23'00222—dc21
DNLM/DLC   98-12094
For Library of Congress   CIP

Contents

Preface

The idea to publish an atlas of the pathology of atherosclerosis and of the clinical manifestations of ischemic heart disease was suggested by Dr. Willis Hurst during my visit to Emory University School of Medicine. He rightly pointed out that clinicians were not always aware of the actual appearance of the arterial lesions they were seeing as angiographic or ultrasound images. This atlas is designed to show practicing clinical cardiologists the reality. It largely illustrates a macroscopic view of coronary artery pathology as seen at autopsy, which has certain inherent drawbacks. The pathologist sees the lesions at only one moment in time, which led to the view that plaques were rather inert lesions. Another drawback is that the pathologist is seeing the worst possible outcome—death. Nevertheless, when autopsy pathology is put into the context of serial angiography, intravascular ultrasound, and angioscopy, a dynamic picture of the disease of atherosclerosis can be constructed.

Microscopy is a personal taste rarely appreciated by practicing clinicians. Illustrations of histology have been kept to a minimum, consistent with describing structure. This atlas is therefore not aimed at providing histopathologists with the minutiae of plaque structure; nor is it aimed at providing the scientist with the latest details on the interactions between the myriad of cytokines, adhesion molecules, and growth factors that are present in plaques. Instead, it is designed to interest the practicing cardiologist, painting a picture with a broad brush of an important disease. While the atlas is broader in scope than is needed by undergraduate students, the principles of the processes are explained without being lost in a wealth of detail.

Dr. Siew Yen Ho has contributed to Chapter 1, on the normal anatomy of human coronary arteries, having had a special interest in this area for many years. The macroscopic pictures of the coronary arteries in this chapter in part appeared previously in a Cordis training and development program developed with Vincent van Ommen and Robert H. Anderson and are used here with their permission.

My own interest, how atherosclerosis produces clinical symptoms, began in 1966, when I joined, in a junior capacity, a team headed by Sir Theo Crawford at St. George's Hospital Medical School. The team included Neville Woolf and W. B. Robertson, who had a major interest in the geographic pathology of atherosclerosis and atherogenesis. Sir Theo was a staunch friend and believer in the work of Duguid, and I was always taught that thrombosis plays a pivotal role in the pathogenesis and clinical expression of ischemic heart disease. Those at St. George's Hospital Medical School never went with the tide of opinion that held thrombosis was a secondary and unimportant phenomenon. The introduction of thrombolysis has now firmly established the role of thrombosis in producing acute infarction. The introduction of effective lipid-lowering agents has opened new vistas. Plaque behavior can be altered; plaques are not static. The role of inflammatory activity within plaques in producing the changes that lead to thrombosis are being recognized. The fact that lipid lowering does not abolish all events has led to a search for other mechanisms, such as infectious agents, as drivers of the plaque inflammatory process. Research into atherosclerosis continues to evolve rapidly.

Over the last 15 years my own research career has been far more within the field of clinical cardiology, in an endeavor to understand how atherosclerosis causes symptoms, rather than in atherogenesis *per se.* Many colleagues both in Europe and in the United States have influenced my thoughts in this regard. My visit to Willis Hurst, Wayne Alexander, and Robert Schlant in Atlanta was a major stimulating event. Over the years, Valentin Fuster, Eric Topol, and Peter Libby have been major influences, although they should not be held responsible for any errors in thought or in fact in this atlas. Anton Becker in Amsterdam has been an example and a source of encouragement.

Michael J. Davies

1

Anatomy of the Coronary Arteries

Siew Yen Ho

INTRODUCTION

The practicing cardiac surgeon or cardiologist needs to know the arrangement of the coronary arteries. Apart from locating and fashioning bypass grafts to the arteries themselves, the surgeon needs to avoid traumatizing the major branches in gaining access to the chambers or valves of the heart. The epicardial courses of the major branches are usually visible on gross inspection, but at times may be deeply buried within epicardial fat. The cardiologist needs to be aware of the aortic origin of the arteries to perform angiography, while an understanding of the epicardial ramifications is crucial information when interpreting angiographic images. Although the overall arrangement of the coronary arteries in the normal heart is well recognized, there remain salient but important variations in origin, arterial dominance, and branching pattern.

CORONARY ARTERY ANATOMY

Origin from Aorta

The normal aortic root is made up of the complex interdigitations between the left ventricular outflow tract and the three aortic sinuses of Valsalva; the leaflets of the aortic valve are supported in semilunar fashion in each of the sinuses (Fig. 1-1). In normal hearts only two of the aortic sinuses give rise to coronary arteries, specifically to the right coronary artery and the main stem of the left coronary artery (Fig. 1-2). This arrangement is very useful for description because, with the heart in its anatomical position, the three aortic sinuses are oriented obliquely relative to the right/left and anterior/posterior coordinates of the body. This makes it difficult to accurately describe the sinuses by standard adjectives, such as right, left, etc. It is an easy matter, however, to designate the aortic sinuses according to whether or not they give rise to a coronary artery. Thus, it is usual to describe the right coronary, left coronary, and noncoronary aortic sinuses. The two aortic sinuses that usually support the coronary arteries are always adjacent to the subpulmonary infundibulum, regardless of whether or not they give rise to a coronary artery. The third sinus is then nonadjacent or nonfacing (Fig. 1-3). In abnormal hearts, therefore, it may be more sensible to describe the sinuses as being the right-hand and left-hand–facing sinuses as viewed from the nonfacing sinus.

Ostial Variations

The arterial orifices are usually positioned just below the sinutubular junction (Fig. 1-4). Examination of several series of presumed normal hearts, however, shows that it is by no means unusual for the coronary arteries to arise at or above the level of the sinutubular junction (1–3) (Fig. 1-5). An orifice arising well above the sinutubular junction, known as "high takeoff," is postulated to be a substrate of sudden cardiac death. This may be due to the initial course of the artery through the aortic wall, with

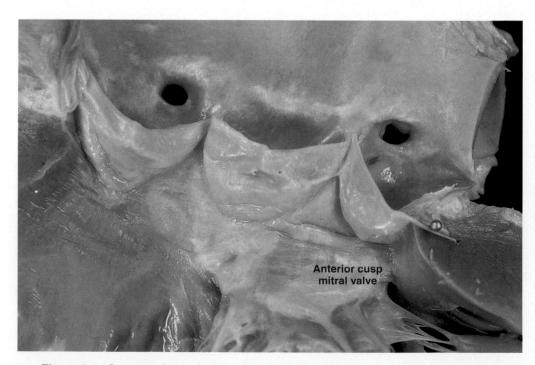

Figure 1-1. Coronary Artery Orifices. This opened aortic root shows how two of the sinuses give rise to coronary arteries and the third does not.

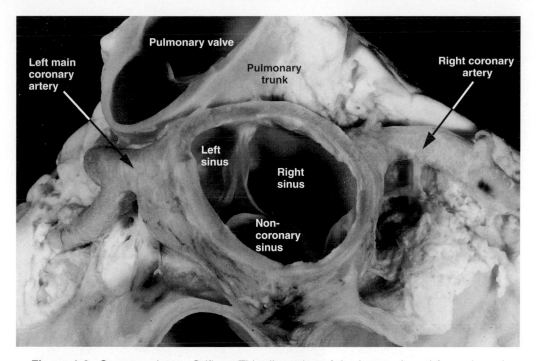

Figure 1-2. Coronary Artery Orifices. This dissection of the heart, viewed from above in anatomical orientation, shows how the coronary arteries arise from the aortic sinuses facing (or adjacent to) the pulmonary trunk. It is more convenient to designate the facing aortic sinuses as the left (L) and right (R) coronary sinuses instead of resorting to spatial coordinates.

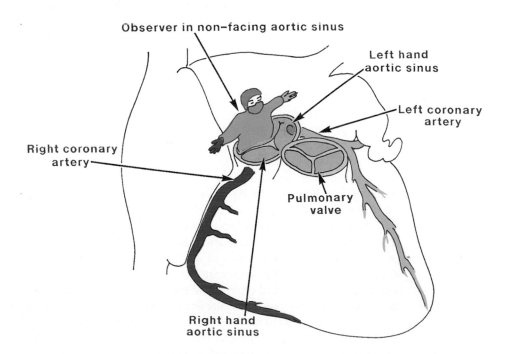

Figure 1-3. Aortic Sinus Nomenclature. Diagram showing the concept of facing aortic sinuses.

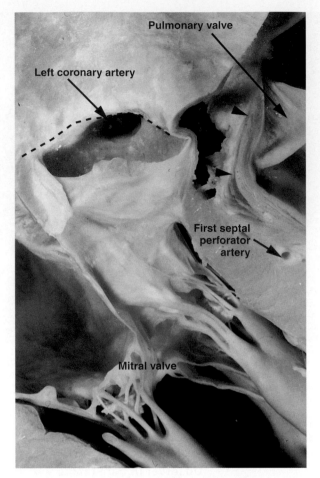

Figure 1-4. Coronary Artery Orifice—Position. This close-up of the left aortic sinus shows the typical origin of a coronary artery adjacent to the sinutubular junction (*arrows*).

the intramural segment producing a funnel effect (4,5). Furthermore, although usually depicted as centrally located in the aortic sinuses, the orifices, especially the orifice of the right coronary artery, tend to be eccentrically positioned (3,6) (Fig. 1-6). Occasionally they are located particularly close to the commissural attachment of an aortic valvar leaflet. The location of the orifice of the right coronary artery close to the zone of apposition between the right and left coronary aortic leaflets becomes important when the aortic root needs to be enlarged using procedures such as the Konno (7) or Rastan and Koncz (8) operations, procedures that require a longitudinal incision to the left of that coronary arterial orifice. It is also possible in apparently normal hearts, even in children, to find an oblique or slit-like course of the artery, or valve-like ridges at its sinusal origin. The significance of these normal variations are unclear, although some studies have linked them to an explained sudden cardiac death (9,10). On rarer occasions, there are more obvious gross variations. Both coronary arteries may arise from one aortic sinus, with one then crossing the commissural attachment of the aortic valvar leaflets to reach its usual location, or there may be a solitary coronary artery. These more abnormal arrangements, as already discussed, have been postulated to be precipitators of sudden death, particularly when one of the coronary arteries then takes a course between aorta and pulmonary trunk having arisen anomalously from the aorta (11). It is in these relatively infrequent circumstances that the nomenclature of right coronary and left coronary aortic sinuses will be potentially misleading. It is exceedingly rare for a coronary artery to arise from the nonadjacent, or nonfacing, aortic sinus (6,12).

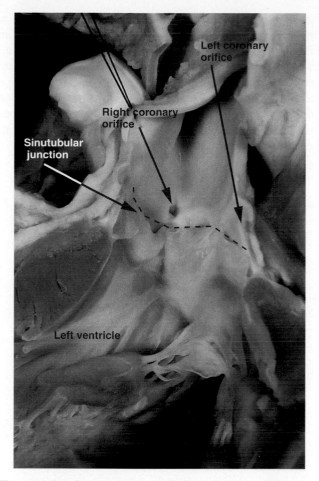

Figure 1-5. Coronary Artery Orifice—Position. This heart has origin of the right coronary artery above the sinutubular junction (*broken line*) and immediately above an aortic valvar commissure.

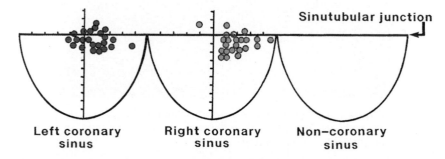

Figure 1-6. Coronary Artery Orifice—Variations. Diagram showing the location of the coronary orifices in a series of 23 normal heart specimens. The luminal aspect of the aorta is displayed. The markers represent tenths of the horizontal and vertical measurements in the sinuses. (Adapted from ref. 3.)

There is further variability in the number of arterial orifices within the aortic sinuses. It is by no means unusual to find the right coronary artery and its infundibular branch taking separate origins from the right coronary aortic sinus (Fig. 1-7). Separate origin of the infundibular artery (described as the "third" coronary artery by some; 13) is more often found in patients over the age of 2 years, suggesting some postnatal modeling of the arterial pattern (14). The sinus nodal artery can also arise directly from the right or the left aortic sinus. It is rare but well recognized to find the anterior interventricular (descending) and circumflex arteries arising from separate orifices within the left coronary aortic sinus.

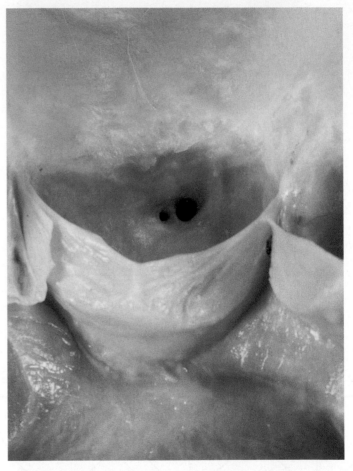

Figure 1-7. Infundibular Artery—Aortic Origin. The infundibular artery arises independently just adjacent to larger right coronary artery.

ANATOMY OF THE EPICARDIAL ARTERIES

The right and left coronary arteries arise from the aorta (Fig. 1-8) and the major branches of these arteries then run within the atrioventricular and interventricular grooves (Fig. 1-9), with division of the left coronary artery into circumflex and anterior interventricular branches producing the three vessels of clinical parlance. Those arteries within the interventricular grooves are then the anterior and posterior descending (or interventricular) arteries. Those within the atrioventricular grooves are the right coronary artery and the circumflex branch of the left coronary artery. The reason for recognizing only these three arteries, rather than all four that occupy the atrioventricular and interventricular grooves, is that there is important variation in the origin of the posterior descending artery. This vessel can arise from either the right coronary artery or from the circumflex artery, thus accounting for the important concept of arterial dominance (Fig. 1-10). Oblique and perpendicular branches from the descending interventricular arteries supply the ventricular wall and the septum. Longitudinal branches springing from the arteries within the atrioventricular grooves either pass upward into the atrial, or downward into the ventricular myocardium. Description of the typical patterns for these branches and their variation is simplified by concentrating on the three major coronary arteries: the right, circumflex, and anterior descending arteries, respectively.

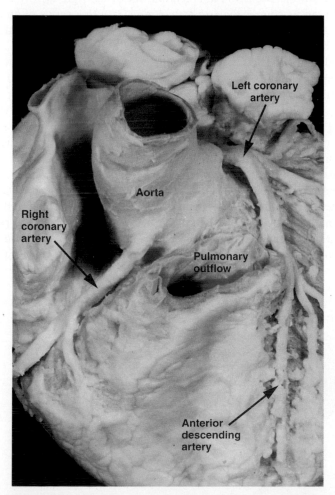

Figure 1-8. Anatomy of Proximal Coronary Arteries. This heart has been prepared by removing the subpulmonary infundibular to show the origin of the coronary arteries from the aortic sinuses.

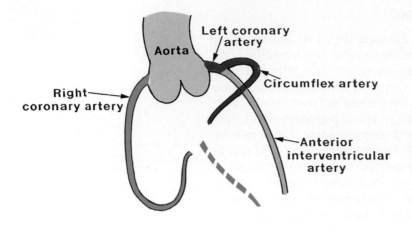

Figure 1-9. Coronary Artery Anatomy. Diagram showing the right, circumflex, and anterior interventricular arteries in their respective grooves as viewed from the frontal aspect. The course of the posterior interventricular artery is indicated by the broken line in blue.

The Right Coronary Artery

The proximal course of the right coronary artery is almost at right angles to the aortic sinus from which it emerges (Fig. 1-2). From this proximal segment, which extends for about 1.5 cm in the adult heart, usually arises an infundibular (conal) branch and the anterior atrial branch. Beyond these branches, the right coronary artery turns to the right and downward as it enters the epicardial fat of the right atrioventricular groove (Fig. 1-11). Along its course, the artery then gives rise to a series of anterior, middle, and posterior atrial arteries that run upward to supply the atrial musculature. In 55% to 66% of individuals, one of these arteries, usually the anterior one, is particularly prominent and forms the artery to the sinus node (15,16). Distal origin of this artery to the sinus node, with a course across the right atrial appendage, is of major importance to the surgeon, since inadvertent damage to the vessel can be the prelude to subsequent disease of the sinus node. Other branches, variable in number, run downward from the right coronary artery to supply the right anterior wall of the ventricle. These are generally called the right anterior ventricular branches. Of these, the infundibular and acute marginal arteries are sufficiently constant to have specific names. Their course is usually short, although one of them, the preventricular branch (7), may extend diagonally across the ventricular wall toward the cardiac apex. Occasionally, an accessory anterior descending (interventricular) artery, as described in the heart of Sir James McKenzie (17), may arise from the proximal portion of the right coronary artery to parallel the interventricular branch arising from the left coronary artery. As the right coronary artery passes along the diaphragmatic surface of the heart, it

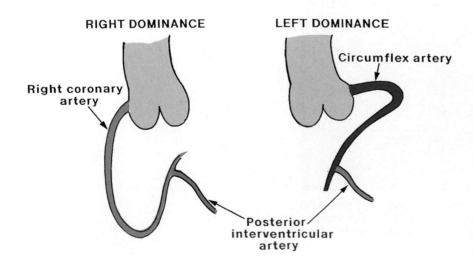

Figure 1-10. Coronary Artery Dominance. The concept of coronary arterial dominance.

reaches the cardiac crux in 90% of individuals, where it gives off the artery to the atrioventricular node and the posterior descending artery (Fig. 1-12). In about 10% of individuals, the left circumflex artery gives rise to the posterior descending artery (Fig. 1-13).

The most commonly used and absolute definition of dominance is the artery right (90%) or left circumflex (10%) that gives rise to the posterior descending and atrioventricular nodal artery. In many subjects who are right-dominant–defined in this way, the right coronary artery continues beyond the crux as the left ventricular branch that supplies the diaphragmatic musculature of the left ventricle and the posteromedial papillary muscles of the mitral valve. There is, however, a more relative usage of the word dominance reflecting the proportion of the left ventricular wall that is supplied by the right or left, respectively (see p. 18).

Main Stem of the Left Coronary Artery

This vessel, having originated from the left-hand–facing aortic sinus, runs a very short course behind the pulmonary trunk, rarely longer than 1 cm, before branching into the circumflex and anterior descending arteries (Fig. 1-14). In contrast to the proximal segment of the right coronary artery, the main stem of the left coronary artery usually dips inferiorly at an angle of 45 degrees to the left aortic sinus. Anomalous origin of the left main stem is of major significance, particularly when the stem, of essence then much longer, runs between the aorta and pulmonary trunk. A short main stem can also pose problems, not only in arteriography and coronary perfusion during valvar replacement, but also in its association with a higher incidence of proximal coronary arterial disease (18).

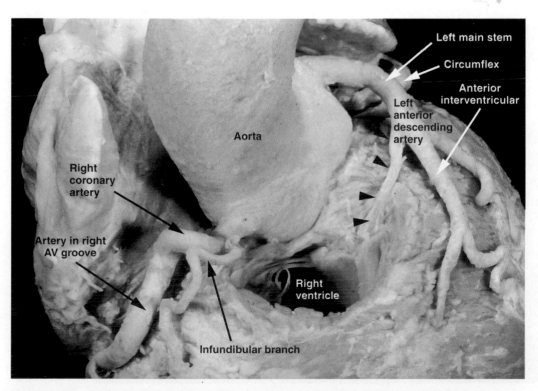

Figure 1-11. Right Coronary Artery. This dissection shows the course of the right coronary artery turning into the right atrioventricular groove. The pulmonary valve has been removed to display the course of the first septal perforating artery (*arrowheads*) from the left anterior descending artery.

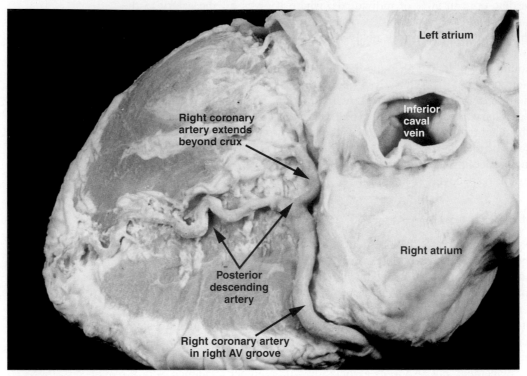

Figure 1-12. Right Dominant Coronary Artery. The right coronary artery supplies the posterior descending artery (right coronary arterial dominance) and continues beyond the cardiac crux to supply the diaphragmatic surface of the left ventricle (*arrow*).

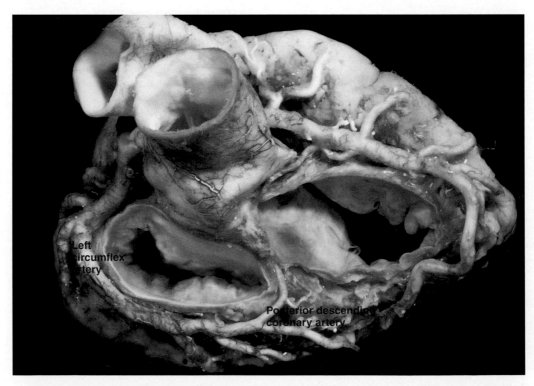

Figure 1-13. Left Coronary Artery Dominance. The atrioventricular grooves are dissected to show the course of the right coronary and left circumflex coronary arteries. The left circumflex artery continues all round the mitral orifice to reach the posterior crux, where it then continues as the posterior descending coronary artery.

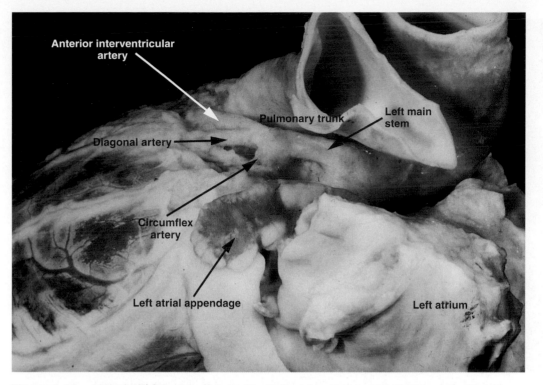

Figure 1-14. Main Left Coronary Artery. The left main stem passes between the pulmonary trunk and the left atrial appendage. It divides to supply anterior interventricular and circumflex branches.

The Anterior Descending Coronary Artery

The branching point of the main stem of the left coronary artery behind the pulmonary trunk is directly related to the anterosuperior end of the ventricular septum. The anterior descending artery, therefore, runs directly into the interventricular groove, giving oblique branches to the musculature of the right and left ventricles, with those branches supplying the left ventricle designated as the diagonal arteries, often described as first, second, and so on (Fig. 1-15). The first diagonal branch, nonetheless, is usually a small branch to the right ventricular infundibulum. In cases of occlusion of the anterior descending coronary artery, this branch may link with its counterpart on the right side to form the ring of Vieussens, which then acts as a collateral circuit. The other crucial branches of the interventricular artery are the septal perforating arteries, which run perpendicularly into the substance of the muscular septum. The first septal perforating artery is the most significant. This prominent artery runs into the septum through the groove, which separates the free-standing subpulmonary infundibulum from the aortic root (Figs. 1-12, 1-15). The artery has a relatively constant relationship to the right-hand–facing leaflet of the pulmonary valve. Knowledge of this relationship should prevent surgical damage to the pulmonary valve should it be required for use in the Ross procedure (19). Additional perforating arteries are variable in number, but we have rarely encountered more than three. Beyond the first diagonal artery, the anterior descending artery often runs intramyocardially for some distance before resurfacing as it approaches the apex. The significance of such myocardial bridging (20) has yet to be fully established. The usual course of the anterior descending artery is then across the apex of the heart, where it turns toward the cardiac base in the posterior interventricular groove. Connections can be established here with branches of the posterior descending (interventricular) artery.

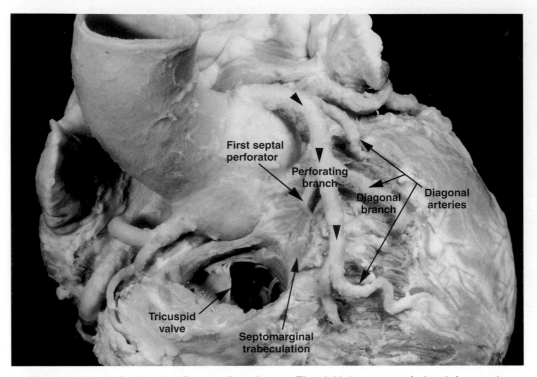

Figure 1-15. Left Anterior Descending Artery. The initial course of the left anterior descending coronary artery (anterior interventricular artery) (*arrowheads*) gives origin to perforating and diagonal branches. Note that the first septal perforating artery passes into the septal musculature behind the anterior limb of the septomarginal trabeculation.

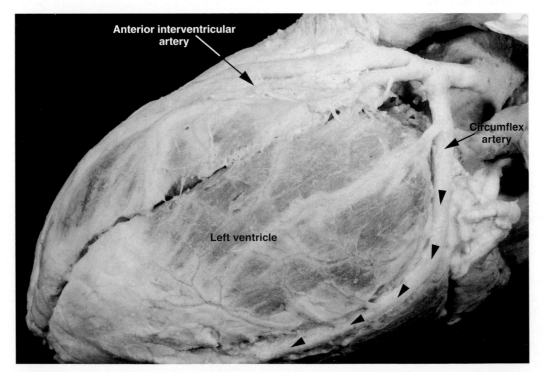

Figure 1-16. Left Circumflex Artery. The circumflex artery in this heart supplies branches to the lateral wall of the left ventricle and terminates as the obtuse or left marginal artery (*arrowheads*).

The Circumflex Coronary Artery

The circumflex artery, having arisen from the main stem of the left coronary artery behind the origin of the pulmonary trunk, passes beneath the left atrial appendage to enter the left atrioventricular groove. Its course varies markedly between individuals. In some the artery is relatively insignificant, supplying merely the obtuse margin of the left ventricle through one or more marginal branches (Fig. 1-16). Often this pattern is seen in the presence of a third major branch arising directly from the left main stem, the so-called "intermediate artery" (Fig. 1-17). In a majority of individuals, perhaps 10%, the circumflex artery is much larger. It then runs throughout the left atrioventricular groove, giving superior branches to the left atrium and marginal branches to the musculature of the left ventricle. With this pattern, known as left dominance (Fig. 1-8), the circumflex artery gives rise at the crux to the posterior descending artery and the artery to the atrioventricular node. It then continues into the right atrioventricular groove to supply part of the diaphragmatic wall of the right ventricle (Fig. 1-18). The course of the circumflex artery within the atrioventricular groove is between the hinge of the mitral valve and the great cardiac vein (Fig. 1-19), placing it at risk of injury during replacement of the mitral valve or during resection of posteriorly located accessory for atrioventricular conduction pathways. It is one of the superior atrial branches of the circumflex artery, which, in 45% of the population, supplies the artery to the sinus node. In a small proportion of individuals, the artery to the sinus

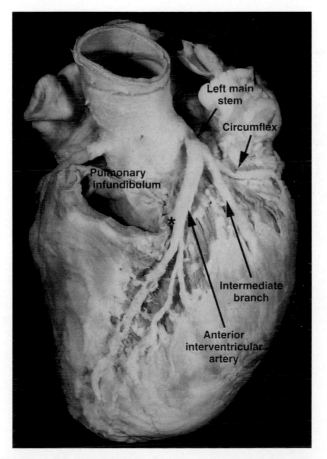

Figure 1-17. Intermediate Coronary Artery. In this heart there is an intermediate branch from the left main stem and a relatively insignificant circumflex artery. Note that the first septal perforating artery (*asterisk*) penetrates behind the subpulmonary infundibulum.

node can arise distally from the circumflex artery, in some instances arising at the crux. As with distal origin from the right coronary artery, this arrangement is mostly of surgical significance.

The Posterior Descending (Interventricular) Artery

As already described, in 90% of individuals this artery is a branch of the right coronary, while in about 10% of persons it is a branch of the circumflex artery (Fig. 1-10). In a small proportion of individuals, the posterior descending artery takes an early origin from the right coronary and runs obliquely across the diaphragmatic surface of the right ventricle. In these cases, the vessel is more readily accessible for grafts using the right internal mammary artery. Regardless of its origin, the artery descends eventually within the posterior interventricular groove. It then gives rise to a series of perforating arteries that run forward in the substance of the muscular septum, often connecting with the perforating branches of the anterior interventricular artery. The posterior descending artery itself usually terminates at the ventricular apex, where again it can connect with the terminal ramifications of the anterior descending artery. In a proportion of individuals, the terminal branches of the circumflex and right coronary arteries descend parallel to either side of the posterior interventricular groove. With this relatively rare, and so-called "balanced," pattern there may not be a true posterior descending coronary artery.

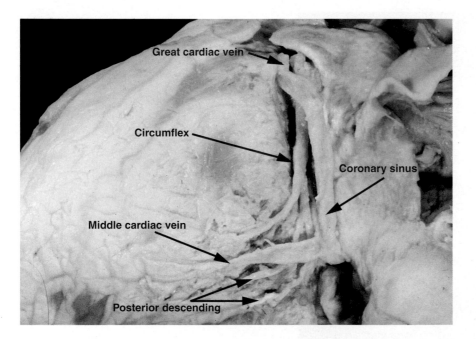

Figure 1-18. Dominant Left Circumflex Artery. This heart illustrates the course of a dominant circumflex artery giving rise to the posterior descending artery. Note its relationship to the cardiac veins.

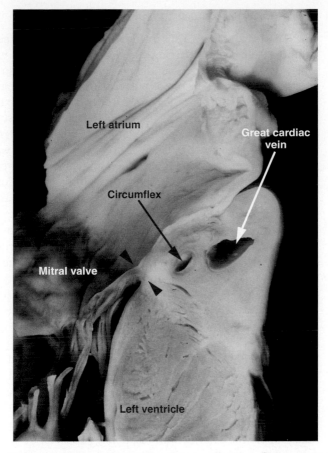

Figure 1-19. Left Circumflex Artery—Position. This section through the posterolateral region of the left atrioventricular junction shows the left coronary circumflex artery lying between the hinge of the mitral leaflet (*between arrowheads*) and the great cardiac vein.

TERMINOLOGY AND ITS PROBLEMS

The arrangement of the major coronary arteries and their branches is of obvious clinical relevance, but problems can arise due to variations in terminology. For instance, the anterior descending coronary artery is also described as the anterior interventricular artery. The major branches of the left coronary artery, the anterior descending and circumflex arteries, are described in some texts as the anterior and posterior divisions, respectively. The intermediate artery has also been labeled as the first diagonal branch of the left coronary artery (21), or the lateral branch (6), the latter designation recognizing its role in supplying the lateral wall of the left ventricle. It is, nonetheless, the concept of arterial dominance that gives most problems. According to the terminology used by the investigators in the Coronary Artery Surgery Study (CASS) (21), and by McAlpine (6), right coronary arterial dominance is described only when the right artery passes beyond the cardiac crux to send branches directly to the diaphragmatic surface of the left ventricle. Other investigators have then added further complications by describing this pattern as "real right dominance" (22). For those who use this convention, the arrangement in which the posterior descending artery is the terminal portion of the right coronary artery is described as a balanced pattern (6,21). The inferior diaphragmatic surface of the left ventricle is then supplied by branches from the circumflex artery. In such hearts, the circumflex artery can also supply the artery to the atrioventricular node, contrary to common belief that the nodal artery always arises from the artery that supplies the posterior descending artery (6). It is also held by many, nonetheless, that the artery that gives rise to the posterior interventricular artery is the dominant one. Thus, there is universal agreement that left coronary arterial dominance refers to the situation in which the circumflex artery supplies the posterior descending coronary artery. The resolution to these problems is to specify the origin of not only the posterior interventricular artery, but also the arteries that supply the inferior wall of the left ventricle.

MICROSTRUCTURE OF THE EPICARDIAL ARTERIES

The coronary arteries have a media banded on the luminal surface by a single substantial elastic lamina, which, as seen in perfused arteries, is not crenellated or wavy. The adventitial aspect of the media is bounded by the external elastic lamina, which is thicker than the internal but again essentially a single structure (Fig. 1-20). The media contains only a few very fine strands of elastic and is predominantly made up of smooth muscle cells embedded in a fine connective tissue matrix. The epicardial coronary arteries are, therefore, adopted to vasoconstriction rather than being purely conductance arteries (Fig. 1-21). When the connective of the vessel wall is displayed the media contains fine collagen, while the adventitia is seen as a thick layer of dense thick collagen bands with high tensile strength (Fig. 1-22).

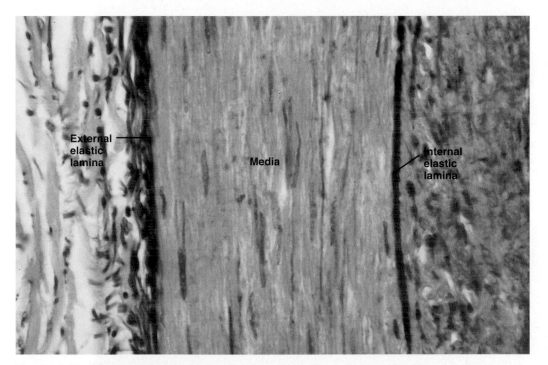

Figure 1-20. Microanatomy of Coronary Artery Wall. The histological section has been stained to show elastic laminae black. The media is bordered on the intimal side by the single internal elastic lamina. The boundary between the media and the adventitia is marked by the external elastic lamina.

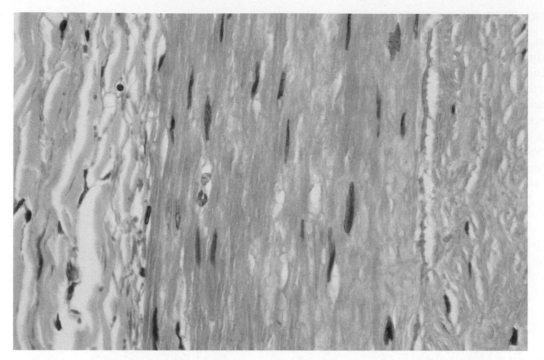

Figure 1-21. Microanatomy of Coronary Artery Wall. The media is made up largely of smooth muscle cells arranged with their long axis and the nuclear long axis circumferentially around the lumen.

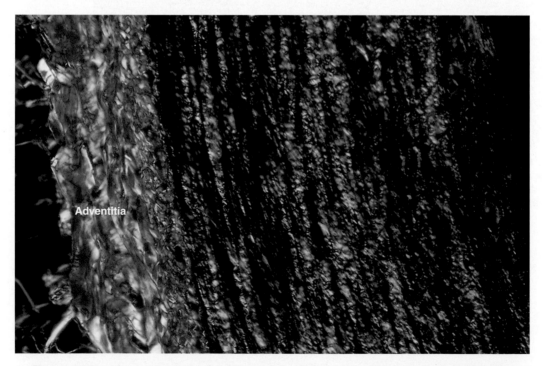

Figure 1-22. Microanatomy of Coronary Artery Wall. In this section stained with the dye Sirius Red viewed under polarized light, fine collagen in the media shows green. The adventitia is a thick band of yellow-red dense collagen. If a vessel wall is tested mechanically the adventitia has by far the greatest tensile strength.

REFERENCES

1. Angelini P. Normal and anomalous coronary arteries: definitions and classification. *Am Heart J* 1989;117: 418–434.
2. Turner K, Navaratnam V. The positions of the coronary arterial osti. *Clin Anat* 1996;9:376–380.
3. Muriago M, Sheppard MN, Ho SY, Anderson RH. The location of the coronary arterial orifices in the normal heart. *Clin Anat* 1997;10:1–6.
4. Bellhouse BJ, Bellhouse FH, Reid KG. Fluid mechanics of the aortic root with application to coronary flow. *Nature* (London). 1968;219:1059–1061.
5. Waller BF, Orr CM, Slack JD, Pinkertan CA, Van Tassel J, Peters T. Anatomy, histology and pathology of coronary arteries: a review relevant to new interventional and imaging techniques. *Clin Cardiol* 1992;15: 451–457.
6. McAlpine WA. *Heart and coronary arteries: anatomical atlas for clinical diagnosis, radiological investigations and surgical treatment.* Berlin: Springer-Verlag, 1986:134.
7. Konno S, Imai Y, Iida T, Nakajima M, Tatsuno K. A new method for prosthetic replacement in congenital aortic stenosis associated with hypoplasia of the aortic valve ring. *J Thorac Cardiovasc Surg* 1975;70:909–917.
8. Rastan H, Koncz J. Aortoventriculoplasty. A new technique for the treatment of left ventricular outflow tract obstruction. *J Thorac Cardiovasc Surg* 1976;71:920–927.
9. Taylor AJ, Rogan KM, Virmani R. Sudden cardiac death associated with isolated congenital coronary artery anomalies. *J Am Coll Cardiol* 1992;20:640–647.
10. Corrado D, Thiene G, Cocco P, Frescura C. Non atherosclerotic coronary artery disease and sudden death in the young. *Br Heart J* 1992;68:601–607.
11. Cheitlin MD, DeCastro CM, McAllister HA. Sudden death as a complication of anomalous left coronary origin from the anterior sinus of Valsalva. *Circulation* 1974;50:780–787.
12. Ishikawa T, Otsuka T, Suzuki T. Anomalous origin of the left main coronary artery from the non coronary sinus of Valsalva [Letter]. *Pediatr Cardiol* 1990;11:173–174.
13. Schlesinger MJ, Zoll PM, Wessler S. The conus artery: a third coronary artery. *Am Heart J* 1949;38:823–838.
14. Edwards BS, Edwards WD, Edwards JE. Aortic origin of conus artery. Evidence of postnatal coronary development. *Br Heart J* 1981;45:555–558.
15. James TN. The sinus node. *Am J Cardiol* 1977;40:965–986.
16. Busquet J, Fontan F, Anderson RH, Ho SY, Davies MJ. The surgical significance of the atrial branches of the coronary arteries. *Int J Cardiol* 1984;6:223–234.
17. Waterston D. Sir James MacKenzie's heart. *Br Heart J* 1939;1:237–248.
18. Saltissi S, Webb-Peploe MM, Coltart DJ. Effects of variation in coronary artery anatomy on distribution of stenotic lesions. *Br Heart J* 1979;42:146–191.
19. Geens M, Gonzalez-Lavin, Dawburn C, Ross DN. The surgical anatomy of the pulmonary root in relation to the pulmonary valve autograft and surgery of the right ventricular outflow tract. *J Thorac Cardiovasc Surg* 1971;62:262–267.
20. Ge J, Erbel R, Rupprecht HJ, Koch L, Kearncy P, Gorge G, Haude M. Meyer J. Comparison of intravascular ultrasound and angiography in the assessment of myocardial bridging. *Circulation* 1994;89:1725–1732.
21. The principal investigators of CASS and their associates. The National Heart, Lung and Blood Institute Coronary Artery Surgery Study (CASS). *Circulation* 1981;63:II-181.
22. Nerantzis CE, Papachristos JCH, Gribizi JE, Voudris VA, Infantis GP, Koroxenidis GT. Functional dominance of the right coronary artery: Incidence in the human heart. *Clin Anat* 1996;9:10–13.

2

Atherosclerosis:
The Process

DEFINITIONS

Pathologists, angiographers, and clinical cardiologists have different perspectives of the disease called atherosclerosis. A definition of what is and what is not atherosclerosis is therefore essential.

Atherosclerosis is an intimal disease of large- to medium-sized arteries including the aorta, carotid, coronary, and cerebral arteries. Within this size range, however, some arterial systems seem very vulnerable, as evidenced by the coronary arteries, while others, such as the internal mammary arteries, are resistant to atherosclerosis. The reasons for this divergence are not known. Intramyocardial arteries less than 1000 μm in external diameter are usually immune.

A very specific feature of atherosclerosis is that it is a focal rather than a diffuse intimal disease. The localized nature of atherosclerosis is best appreciated in cross sections of the coronary artery, where one portion of the vessel wall is abnormal but there is also a segment of normal vessel wall (Figs. 2-1, 2-2). Each individual lesion in the intima, known as a plaque, contains a connective tissue matrix including collagen, elastin, and proteoglycans produced by smooth muscle cells (Table 2-1). Within the plaque there is also extracellular lipid and lipid contained within cells with a foamy vacuolated cytoplasm, the majority of which can be identified as macrophages by the use of immunohistochemistry. Within the plaque there are also T-lymphocytes and some basophils (mast cells).

Attempts in animals to reproduce a disease resembling all the components of human atherosclerosis are successful only if plasma lipids are raised either by very high fat diets or by genetic defects in lipid metabolism, such as in the Watanabe rabbit. This fact, plus the very strong epidemiological evidence from human disease that high lipid levels are the major risk factor for atherosclerosis, points to the disease being a response to damage in the arterial wall caused by lipid being deposited (1).

In a disease as complex as atherosclerosis there will always be some divergence from these basic definitions. One component of atherosclerosis is smooth muscle proliferation followed by connective tissue matrix deposition. In animal models, intimal injury with endothelial denudation, usually induced by inflating a balloon within an artery, is followed by localized smooth muscle proliferation to form a plaque. The lesion does not, however, reproduce the plaques so typical of human disease unless there is concomitant elevation of the plasma lipids. Isolated smooth muscle proliferation is not atherosclerosis, but the ubiquitous repair response to intimal injury.

In a similar manner, postangioplasty stenosis is caused by the response to intimal tearing and not the disease of atherosclerosis itself.

Diffuse intimal smooth muscle cell proliferation with some localized accentuation at branching points occurs in human coronary arteries with age and is an adaptive response to flow and pressure rather than being atherosclerosis (2,3). The appearance of smooth muscle cells and intimal humps in human coronary arteries is ubiquitous in infants. While sometimes the presence of this intimal fibromuscular thickening is used to suggest that atherosclerosis has already developed in infants, it is more likely to be a simple adaptive change to flow. The existence of smooth muscle cells within the intima of normal human coronary arteries may, however, indicate a susceptibility to atherosclerosis. In human coronary arteries there is no need for migration of smooth muscle cells into the intima from the media to initiate plaque formation; this contrasts

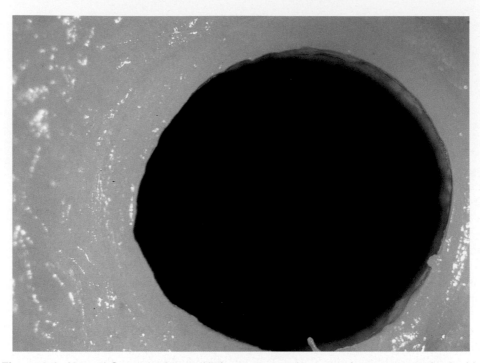

Figure 2-1. Normal Coronary Artery. All the macroscopic views of coronary arteries in this atlas are taken from human perfused fixed necropsy specimens. The lumen has been distended at a pressure of 100 mm Hg with 10% formal saline. In this normal artery the ratio of the wall thickness (intima–media) relative to the lumen can be appreciated. Perfused fixed arteries correspond to the lumen dimensions pertaining at maximal vasodilation *in vivo* and the internal elastic lamina is fully expanded.

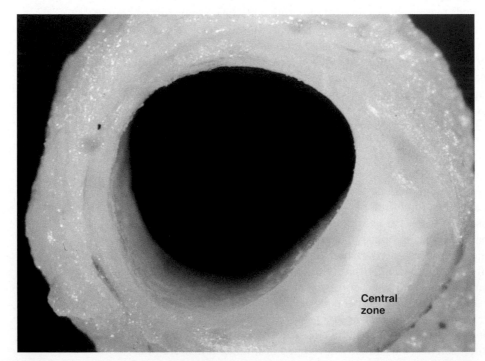

Figure 2-2. Early Coronary Atherosclerosis. The plaque is an eccentrically situated thickening in the intima and has a central zone containing yellow lipid (American Heart Association type IV plaque). Opposite the plaque there is a segment of normal arterial wall and the lumen is not reduced in size. In arteries fixed by perfusion at 100 mm Hg pressure the lumen is approximately round in shape.

Table 2-1. *Constituents of plaques*

Cells
  Macrophages (MØ), smooth muscle cells (SMC), T-lymphocytes, mast cells
Lipid
  Extracellular
  Intracellular—foam cells, mostly MØ
Matrix
  Collagen
  Elastin   Produced by SMC
  Proteoglycan

with smaller animals, where the intima does not normally contain smooth muscle cells.

In the majority of subjects with atherosclerosis there will be a proportion of plaques in which the lesion is almost entirely fibrous and without a significant lipid component. The ways in which such fibrous plaques may arise is uncertain. One view is that they represent the final evolutionary stage of a plaque that once had contained lipid, another view is that there are pathways of plaque initiation and evolution that are not lipid dependent.

Finally, while small arteries are generally immune from atherosclerosis in very severe hyperlipidemia and diabetes, intramyocardial arteries in the range of 400 to 800 μm may develop diffuse intimal thickening containing lipid-filled foam cells.

It is conceptually important to keep native coronary artery atherosclerosis, postangioplasty stenosis, transplant vascular disease, and vein graft disease as distinct entities. These conditions all share some pathological processes, but the mix of lipid accumulation, smooth muscle proliferation, and immune activation differs markedly.

ATHEROSCLEROSIS: PLAQUE MORPHOLOGY

While not easily appreciated or relevant to those more at home with angiograms, the methods of examining atherosclerosis used by pathologists have led to important concepts. The traditional pathology method of examining atherosclerosis has been to slit an artery open longitudinally and view the intimal surface enface. Three types of lesions are found. Fatty streaks or dots (Figs. 2-3, 2-4) are small (up to 4 mm in diameter), yellow, and barely raised above the surface. Raised fibrolipid plaques (Figs. 2-5, 2-6) are elevated above the surface and oval in shape, parallel to the long axis of the artery. The color of fibrolipid plaques varies from all shades of yellow to white, depending on the proportions of lipid to collagen in that particular plaque. Fibrolipid plaques in the aorta, carotid, or femoral arteries may be up to 3 cm in length. Finally, naked-eye examination will reveal plaques covered by thrombus usually designated as complicated lesions (Fig. 2-7).

It is perhaps worth reminding those who pass catheters up from the femoral artery that up to half of subjects over 50 years of age with ischemic heart disease will have an abdominal aorta with mural thrombus comparable to that in Fig. 2-7.

The proportion of the intimal surface of the coronary arteries and aorta covered by these three types of lesion is an indication of the extent of atherosclerosis in that individual, but it is a measurement that can be made only at autopsy. Comparative studies of large autopsy populations with different risk factors, geographic origin, or race (4–6) have shown two important facts about atherosclerosis. First, that in any geographic population the extent of atherosclerosis correlates with the risk of clinically expressed coronary disease in that population. Such epidemiological studies do not, however, imply that there are not unlucky individuals who die from an isolated plaque in a key position, such as the main left coronary artery. It is a supreme example of the

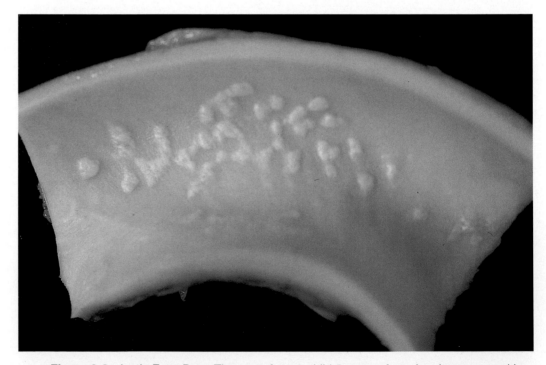

Figure 2-3. Aortic Fatty Dots. The aorta from a child 5 years of age has been opened longitudinally and pinned out flat to allow the intimal surface to be viewed enface. On the intimal surface are a series of yellow dots that barely project above the surface. No advanced plaques are present.

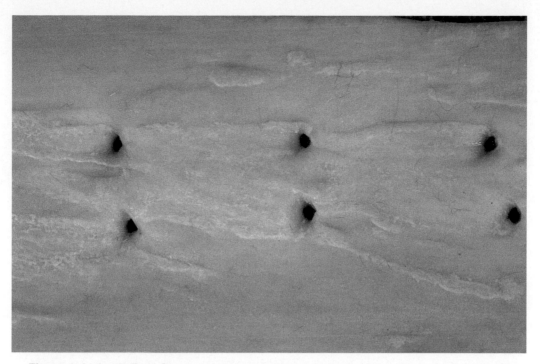

Figure 2-4. Aortic Fatty Streaks. In this aorta from a 20-year-old man there are a series of yellow streaks that are only just raised above the intimal surface. While a great deal is often made of the lesions being related to flow dividers, i.e., intercostal artery orifices, as can be seen here most fatty streaks bear no relation to branch points.

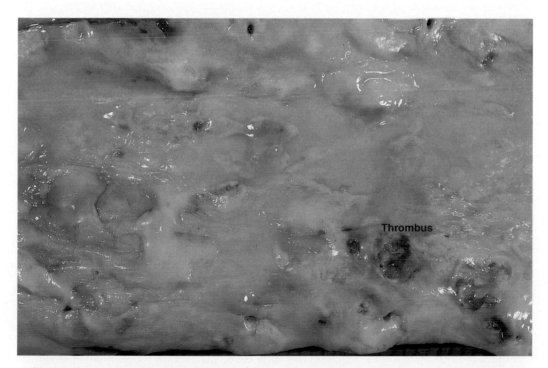

Figure 2-5. Aorta-Fibrolipid Plaques. On the intimal surface there are a range of plaque types. Some are fatty streaks, others are raised more above the surface and are bigger. These larger plaques are raised fibrolipid lesions. The largest are white in color due to the presence of a large amount of collagen. Other raised plaques are yellow due to their high content of lipid. One plaque has developed thrombus on the surface.

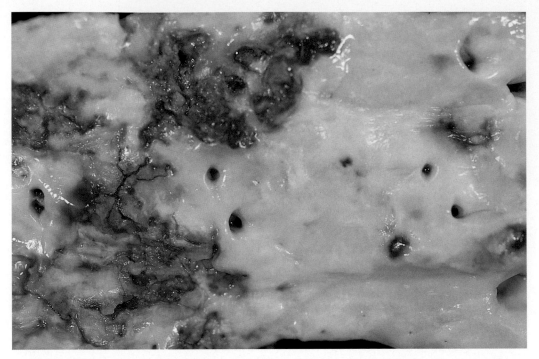

Figure 2-6. Aorta-Complicated Plaques. There are some intact raised plaques on the intima but the majority of the plaques have undergone disruption (ulceration) and are covered by thrombus.

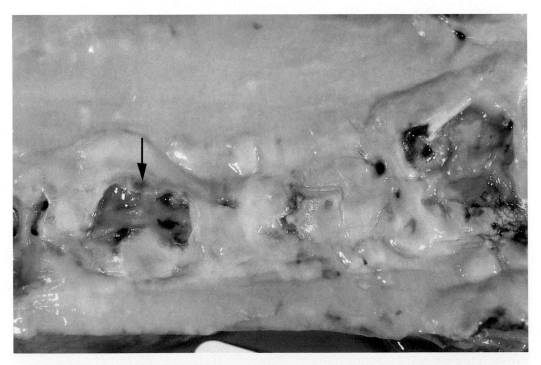

Figure 2-7. Ulcerated Aortic Plaques. Two large raised plaques each over 1 cm in length have undergone ulceration. In one (*arrow*) the lipid core has washed away, leaving a crater that is beginning to be recovered by intimal growth. The other still has an exposed lipid core covered by thrombus. In the carotid artery this type of plaque is strongly associated with transient cerebral ischemic attacks due to platelet emboli.

aphorism that epidemiology reveals a lot about populations and nothing about individuals. Second, many of the risk factors known to be linked to clinically expressed coronary disease operate in part by increasing the total number of plaques (7). For example, on a population basis, smokers have more coronary and aortic plaques than nonsmokers. Similar data exists for hyperlipidemia, hypertension, and diabetes.

Far more detailed morphological studies of plaques have been made involving histology, immunohistochemistry, and scanning electron microscopy. These have culminated in a detailed staging of plaques published by the American Heart Association (2) (Fig. 2-8). Studies that look at different age cohorts of individuals dying of noncardiac disease have allowed a scheme to be drawn up that gives a perspective on how plaques evolve.

Stage I is essentially a preatherosclerotic lesion and consists of the adhesion of monocytes to the intact endothelial surface followed by their migration into the intima (Figs. 2-9, 2-10).

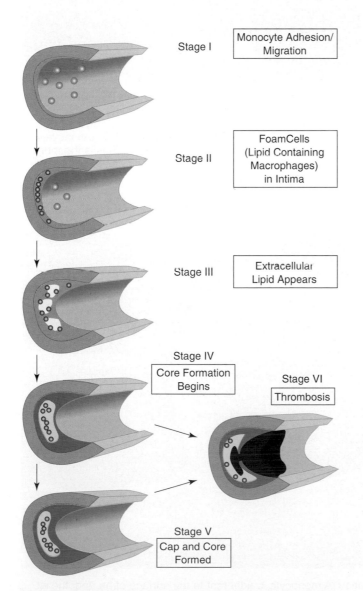

Stage I — Monocyte Adhesion/ Migration

Stage II — FoamCells (Lipid Containing Macrophages) in Intima

Stage III — Extracellular Lipid Appears

Stage IV — Core Formation Begins

Stage V — Cap and Core Formed

Stage VI — Thrombosis

Figure 2-8. The American Heart Association Plaque Nomenclature. The schema provides both a nomenclature and a proposed evolutionary path for plaque formation.

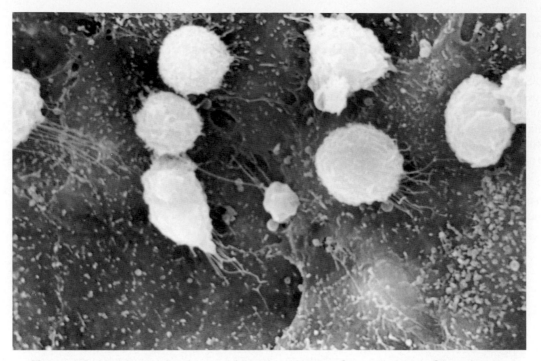

Figure 2-9. Monocyte Adhesion and Migration—Human Coronary Artery. Several monocytes are adherent to the endothelial surface (scanning electron microscopy). In scanning electron microscopy the vessel is perfused with a fixative (glutaraldehyde) and then the endothelial surface can be viewed enface at very high magnifications. The monocytes appear to be attached to the surface of the endothelial cell by fine strands. This is the morphological expression of reaction between adhesion molecules expressed on the surface of the endothelial cell and their ligands on the monocyte.

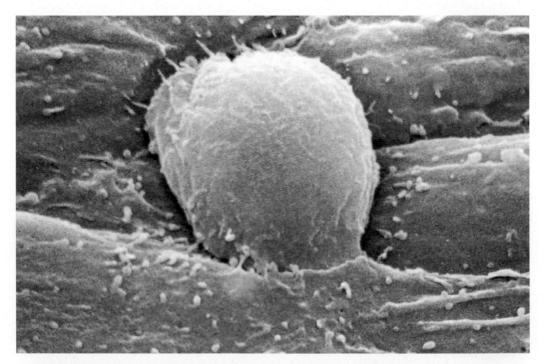

Figure 2-10. Monocyte Migration. A monocyte is adherent to the surface of an endothelial cell and is beginning to insert itself between two adjacent endothelial cells (scanning electron microscopy).

Stage II is the fatty streak or dot and consists of a focal accumulation of lipid-filled macrophages (foam cells) in the intima (Fig. 2-11). The overlying endothelium is intact. Some T-lymphocytes are also present. Fatty streaks are, however, not heterogeneous in their makeup; a small proportion of fatty streaks are predominantly made up from lipid-filled smooth muscle cells.

Stage III has the appearance of extracellular lipid in addition to that contained within foam cells, and smooth muscle cell numbers have increased.

Stage IV has the extracellular lipid coalescing into the center of the plaque and a layer of smooth muscle cell forms over the lipid core just beneath the endothelial surface.

Stage Va has a fully formed lipid core with an acellular mass of cholesterol, some of which is in the crystalline form. There is a well-developed cap of fibrous tissue separating the core from the lumen (Figs. 2-12, 2-13). The margins of the core are lined by lipid-filled foam cells of macrophage origin.

Stage Vb has the features of Va but also has calcification. Plaques of type **Vc** are solid and fibrous without a lipid core (Fig. 2-14) and a very minor macrophage content.

Stage VI are plaques complicated by thrombosis.

This proposed sequence of plaque evolution has much to recommend it but some facets remain uncertain. The scheme tends to obscure the fact that type Va plaques, even within one individual, cover a wide spectrum with regard to the size of the lipid core, the cap thickness, the number of macrophages present, and the density of smooth muscle cells in the cap. The origin of type Vc plaques is uncertain. Some may represent healing of plaques complicated by thrombus; other plaques have a uniform structure suggesting they were fibrous from the start. The presence of lesions at all stages in one adult aorta suggests that the sequence of plaque evolution is initiated throughout life. Studies of cohorts at different ages in subjects who die from accidents sug-

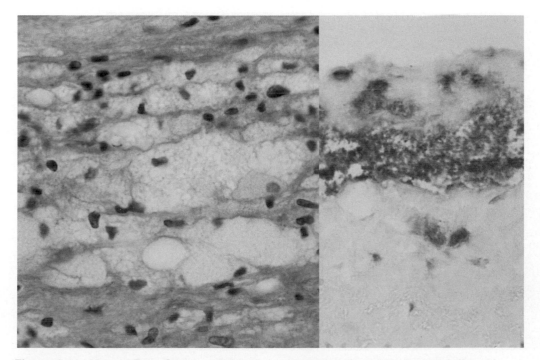

Figure 2-11. Human Fatty Streak—Histology. In conventionally stained hematoxylin and eosin, histological sections of foam cells are large and have a clear slightly granular cytoplasm. Immunohistochemistry is a technique in which antibodies to known antigens are applied to the histological section. The antibody is tagged with an enzyme (phosphatase) to produce a red product allowing binding to be recognized. The antibody used here was to the macrophage antigen CD68 and the red signal allows the foam cells to be recognized as being macrophages.

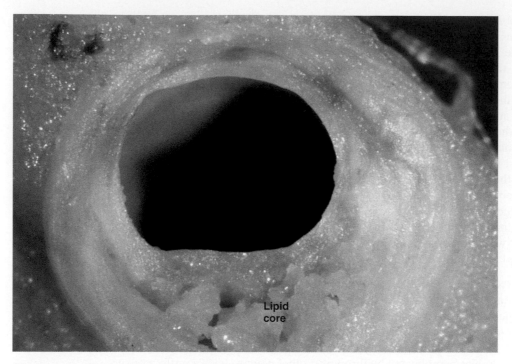

Figure 2-12. Stage Va Coronary Plaque. There is a large lipid core within the plaque. The core consists of crumbling yellow lipid material. The core is separated from the lumen of the artery by a gray-white fibrous cap rich in collagen. Opposite the plaque there is a segment of normal arterial wall.

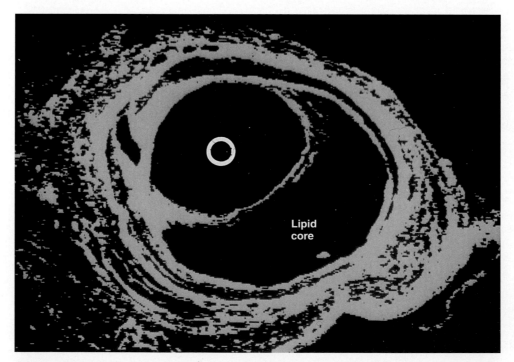

Figure 2-13. Stage Va Coronary Plaque. The collagen has been imaged by binding with the dye Sirius Red and then the signal converted to a yellow image. The plaque has a lipid core that is devoid of collagen. The plaque cap varies markedly in thickness. The lumen has been marked with an O. The artery wall has a clear circumferential zone, which is the media. The image is very similar to those obtained by intravascular ultrasound.

gest that the transition from fatty streaks, which first appear in children, to type Va plaques, which appear in the 20- to 30-year-old age group is a lengthy process. It is, however, not known if the progression accelerates with age or is at a uniform rate for all plaques in an individual. There is good evidence from comparative studies of different geographic populations that not all fatty streaks progress, and some may indeed regress and vanish (8). The number of fatty streaks present in children in populations such as the South African Bantu is high, yet study of adults from the same population shows few later-stage plaques.

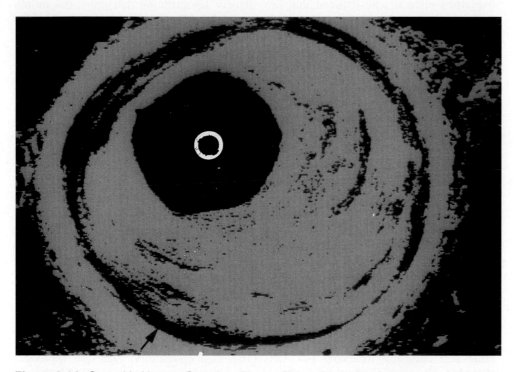

Figure 2-14. Stage Vc Human Coronary Plaque. The collagen has been imaged to show the collagen in a manner identical to Fig. 13. The plaque is solid without a lipid core. The lumen is marked with an O. The media (*arrow*) is a translucent zone due to its low collagen content.

ATHEROSCLEROSIS: THE INITIATION PHASE

The earliest human lesion that can be recognized by naked-eye and histological examination is the fatty streak with a predominant cell population of lipid-filled macrophages. In animal models of atherosclerosis, an earlier stage can be recognized by scanning electron microscopy—this is the adhesion of blood monocytes to an intact endothelial surface (9). Monocytes then migrate into the intima and become converted to macrophages, which take up lipid to become foam cells (Fig. 2-15). There was an apparent paradox in these findings because macrophages do not have the usual low-density lipoprotein (LDL) receptor allowing them to take up lipid. The paradox was explained once it was realized that low density lipoproteins that enter the intima undergo a series of modifications (10). These modifications first produce a minimally modified product that acts as a proinflammatory mediator (11) and then further modification produces a product recognized by a number of scavenger receptors expressed on the surface of macrophages. These receptors allow macrophage uptake of modified oxidized LDL and at least one has the additional property of not downregulating, allowing the macrophage cytoplasm to become totally distended by lipid forming a foam cell. The demonstration of the existence of a scavenger receptor on macrophages by Brown and Goldstein in 1983 (12) has been followed by the recognition that two isoforms exist of scavenger receptor A (13) and that there are other receptors capable of binding to oxidized lipid, including scavenger receptor B (CD36) (14) and macrosialin (CD68). Animal models in which scavenger receptor A (SAA) is knocked out develop less atherosclerosis (15) than normal mice when challenged, but can form macrophage foam cells, thus confirming that more than one receptor exists for oxidized lipid. A small amount of lipid is taken up by smooth muscle cells via an LDL receptor and possibly a scavenger receptor, but although lipid droplets appear in the cytoplasm, the degree does not reach the level at which true foam cells are formed.

The cycle of monocyte adhesion, monocyte migration into the intima, conversion to macrophages, fixation in the tissue, division, and activation to produce further inflammatory mediators is mediated by a complex system of cytokines and adhesion molecules. Modified LDL acts to invoke the expression of three adhesion molecules that have ligands on monocytes. These are intercellular adhesion molecule (ICAM), vascular cell adhesion molecule (VCAM) (16), and endothelial adhesion molecule (ELAM). Chemotactic factors, such as monocyte chemotactic factor (MCP-1), are induced, which initiate the migration. The viability division and expression of scavenger receptors on monocytes in the intima depends on local production of macrophage colony stimulating factor (MCSF-1) (17–19). The creation of a fatty streak, therefore, involves complex cell interactions. The endothelial cell layer is structurally intact over fatty streaks.

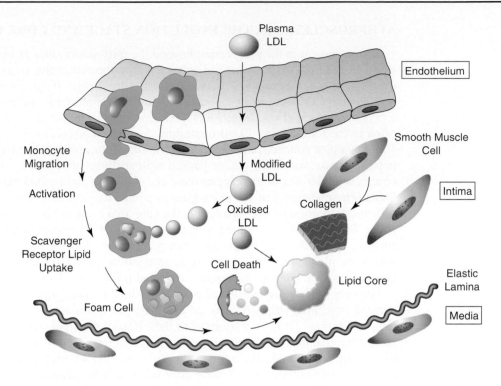

Figure 2-15. The Basic Processes in Atherosclerosis. Plasma low-density lipoprotein (LDL), which has entered the intima, becomes modified and induces changes in the endothelium leading to monocyte migration. Within the intima further oxidation of LDL leads to a form that is actively taken up by macrophages to form foam cells. Macrophage death releases lipid to form the core. Growth factors released by endothelial cells and macrophages stimulate smooth muscle growth and connective tissue matrix synthesis.

ATHEROSCLEROSIS: THE EVOLUTION STAGE AND CORE CREATION

A key element in the progression beyond the fatty streak stage is the appearance of extracellular lipid. At first this is dispersed within the connective tissue matrix as fine droplets, but then begins to coalesce to form a lipid core. By the time plaques have reached stage IV, the core is acellular and contains cholesterol and its esters, often in a crystalline form (Figs. 2-16, 2-17). Oxidized lipid is abundant within the core (20), often in the form of ring-like protein lipid complexes (ceroid) (21). Initially the core still contains a connective tissue matrix but this often vanishes by stage Va, leaving a potential space within the plaque packed with acellular lipid debris. The center of the core is acellular, but at its margins there are numerous lipid-filled macrophages (Fig. 2-18). The phenotype of the macrophages within the core area varies widely. A significant proportion of macrophages in the core area express Tissue Factor, much in an active form, and this combined with the presence of fragments of collagen and lipid surfaces on which blood coagulation can occur makes the core the most thrombogenic part of the plaque (22,23). Tissue Factor production and activation within plaques may be induced from macrophages due to oxidized lipid or to CD40 ligand binding (24).

The origin of the extracellular lipid within the core is regarded in major part to be derived from lipid released from the cytoplasm of macrophage foam cells following their death (Fig. 2-19). A proportion of the extracellular lipid, however, may not have passed through the macrophage but derived from alteration of LDL that became bound to proteoglycans within the intima (25). The cause of the macrophage death is partly due to necrosis initiated by the direct cytotoxicity of lipid peroxides and partly by apoptosis (26–28). In this latter process in which the macrophage is induced to self-destruct by synthesizing enzymes that cleave deoxyribonucleic acid (DNA) in the nucleus, there must be a trigger. One such trigger would be a reduction in the macrophage growth factors such as macrophage-colony stimulating factor-1 (17), on which continuing cell viability depends.

The destruction of the connective tissue matrix in the core area is a key element of the evolution toward a type Va plaque, but is imperfectly understood. A wide range of metalloproteinases capable of breaking down the connective tissue matrix proteins are produced within plaques by activated macrophages (29). The collagen at the margin of a lipid core has a sharply defined edge, suggesting it is created by an active process rather than the tissues simply being pushed apart.

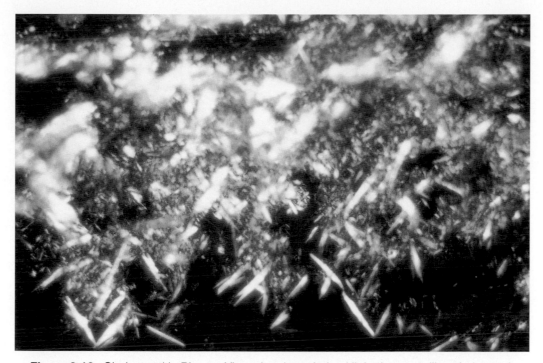

Figure 2-16. Cholesterol in Plaque. Viewed under polarized light the crystalline cholesterol in the core is brightly refringent. Many of the crystals are needle- or boat-shaped.

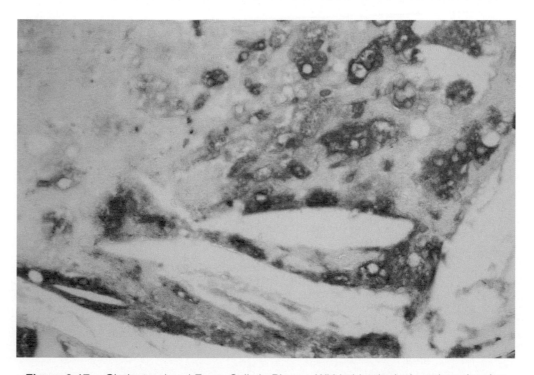

Figure 2-17. Cholesterol and Foam Cells in Plaque. Within histological sections the cholesterol is dissolved out in the processing but their original presence can be recognized by boat-shaped oval spaces in the tissue. The section has been stained by immunohistochemistry for CD68 and all the cells are foam cells of macrophage type.

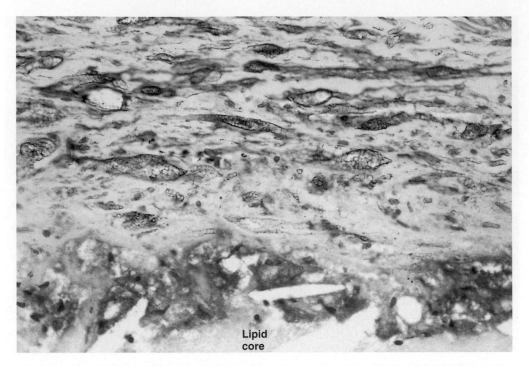

Figure 2-18. Cell Constituents of Plaque Cap. The section has been stained by immuno-histochemistry for CD68 (*red*) indicating macrophages and smooth muscle actin (*brown*). The cap contains mainly smooth muscle cells, some vacuolated due to lipid in the cytoplasm. At the margin of the lipid core the cells are macrophage foam cells.

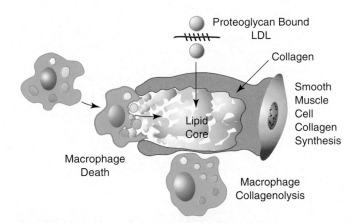

Figure 2-19. Core Creation in the Plaque. The acellular core of lipid is created in part by lipid released from the death of macrophage foam cells, but also in part from low-density lipoprotein particles that have become bound to proteoglycans in the intima. Smooth muscle cells produce collagen to encapsulate and limit the lipid core. Macrophage activity via metalloproteinases destroys collagen to enlarge the core area.

ENDOTHELIAL STATUS OVER PLAQUES

Clear distinction must be made between abnormalities of endothelial function in which the endothelial surface is structurally intact but the production of nitric oxide by endothelial cells is inhibited or, for example, when adhesion molecules, such as VCAM, are expressed and denudation injury in which subendothelial matrix and, in particular, collagen and Von Willebrand factor are exposed to platelets in the blood. There is ample evidence that in atherosclerosis there are functional abnormalities in endothelial cells that may be focal, i.e., over a developing plaque itself or generalized and found in arteries that do not themselves have plaques. The initial phase of monocyte migration is dependent on focal alterations in endothelial expression of adhesion molecules. In subjects with atherosclerosis there is an increase in the responses to vasoconstrictor agents and a marked attenuation of endothelial-dependent relaxation to vasodilating agents (30–32). These changes may be very focal, i.e., related to a specific arterial segment, implying that a plaque is present or there is very widespread occurrence at an early or preatheromatous stage of disease. The endothelial dysfunction has been linked to hypercholesterolemia itself, implying that specific components of cholesterol, such as circulating lipid peroxides, are responsible (33).

In early atherosclerosis (Fig. 2-20) there is no denudation and therefore platelets play no role in plaque initiation. However, once plaques have formed and when monocyte accumulation is advanced, endothelial breaks appear and platelet–vessel wall interaction begins (34,35) (Fig. 2-21). The importance of endothelial denudation is that it allows interaction of the platelet 1a/1b receptor with exposed matrix proteins, leading in turn to activation of the IIb/IIIa receptor binding platelets to platelets via fibrinogen (Fig. 2-22).

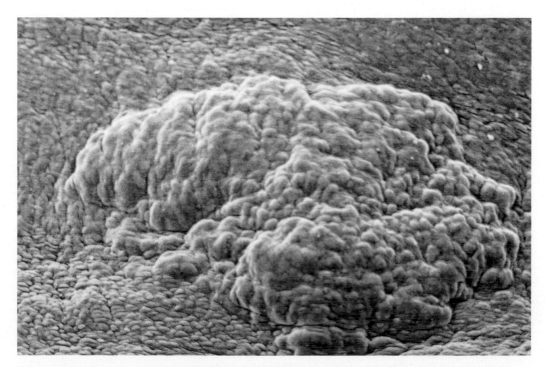

Figure 2-20. Human Fatty Streak. The endothelium viewed by scanning electron microscopy is intact over the intimal lesion.

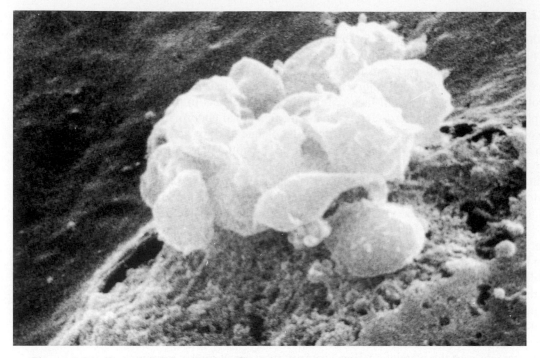

Figure 2-21. Endothelial Denudation. Over this plaque a single endothelial cell has been lost. In this very discrete area a small platelet thrombus has formed. No platelets have adhered to adjacent intact endothelial cells.

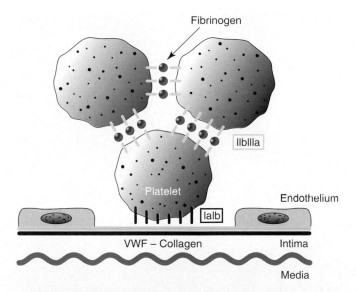

Figure 2-22. Platelet Vessel Wall Interaction. If the endothelium is denuded collagen and Von Willebrand Factor are exposed and a monolayer of platelets adhere because of interaction with the Ia/Ib group of receptors. Platelet-to-platelet interaction is via the IIb/IIIa receptor using fibrinogen as the binder. Von Willebrand factor and fibronectin receptors also play a role in platelet-to-platelet adhesion.

SMOOTH MUSCLE PROLIFERATION COLLAGEN AND THE PLAQUE

From infancy the human coronary intima contains smooth muscle cells. This contrasts to many smaller animals where smooth muscle cells are absent from the intima; smooth muscle cells would therefore have to migrate from the media before a plaque could form. The human coronary intima cannot be said to have atherosclerosis in infancy but the human coronary artery may be primed for plaque formation in later life (36).

All plaques contain smooth muscle cells that produce the connective tissue matrix, consisting predominantly of collagen without which the plaque would disintegrate. The layer of smooth muscle cells in the depths of a plaque at the intimal medial junction are the residue of the original adaptive intimal thickening that develops with age in human coronary arteries (2). Atherosclerosis develops superficial to this layer. Once a lipid core has formed, the collagen within the cap is organized into a regular lattice within which there are lacunae (oval spaces) containing smooth muscle cells that produce and maintain the connective tissue matrix (Fig. 2-23).

A bewildering variety of growth factors initiate and control smooth muscle migration proliferation and their production of matrix proteins (Fig. 2-24), which are rate limiting or dominant is uncertain. All the cell types present within plaques, including smooth muscle cells themselves, produce such growth factors (37). Some of the factors initiate smooth muscle migration or division or synthesis of connective tissue matrix; many have more than one of these functions. Most factors are tested *in vivo* on smooth muscle cells in culture and it is less certain whether the factors act in the same way *in vivo*. Smooth muscle cells have receptors for the growth factors. Some factors modulate collagen synthesis [transforming growth factor-β (TGF-β)], others will suppress connective tissue synthesis (interferon-τ). The growth factors released after acute medial injury, i.e., angioplasty, may differ from those operating with the plaque in primary atherogenesis. It can be assumed that in many plaques smooth muscle proliferation is coupled with macrophage activity and lipid accumulation and the two are in some form of dynamic balance. The creation of a solid fibrous plaque could represent a final stage in which smooth muscle cell proliferation and collagen formation totally predominate. Smooth muscle cell migration into the intima from the media is not a prerequisite of plaque formation, since the human coronary intima from infancy has a population of smooth muscle cells. The arterial response to severe injury, such as occurs during angioplasty where the intimal tear often extends into the media, will, however, also involve migration of medial smooth muscle cells into the intima.

Research into the growth factors modulating the repair process has been prolific, using both smooth muscle cells in culture and animal models where balloon injury causes endothelial denudation and intimal injury. The most widely studied factor so far is platelet-derived growth factor (PDGF), so named because it was found to be stored in platelet granules. In fact, it is also produced by virtually all the cell types present in plaques (38). PDGF, in fact, is two separate gene products PDGF-A and PDGF-B chains. These two products form their covalent dimers AA, BB, AB. There are also separate receptors, PDGFαR and PDGFβR, leading to considerable complexity, where a cell expressing both receptors will respond to all three PDGF dimers, a cell expressing α- and β-receptors will bind PDGF-AB and BB and a cell with only the β-receptor will bind only PDGF-B. Experimental evidence so far suggests that PDGF-B is the major element in the response to arterial injury and antibodies to it, its receptor or antisense oligos will block smooth muscle proliferation (39). Basic fibroblast growth factor (bFGF) is another well-characterized factor that is stored as a complex bound to proteoglycans on the basement membrane of cells and on extracellular connective tissue matrixes. Any injury causes release of the factor with a potent mitogenic affect on smooth cells (40). Antibodies against bFGF will also inhibit injury-induced smooth muscle cell proliferation (41).

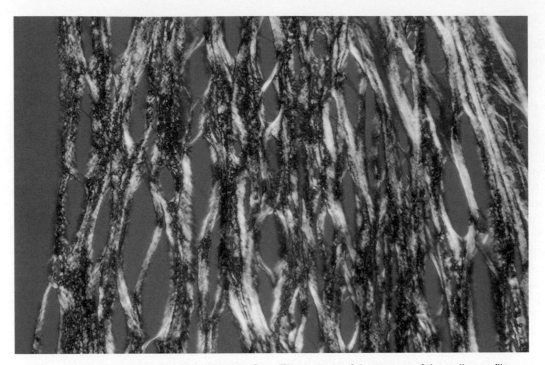

Figure 2-23. Organization of The Plaque Cap. The pattern of the weave of the collagen fibrils can be seen by linking collagen to the dye Sirius Red and examining the tissue by polarized light microscopy. The cap collagen is arranged in a regular interlocking weave pattern suggesting an adaptation toward high tensile strength. Within the oval spaces in the tissue, smooth muscle cells are present.

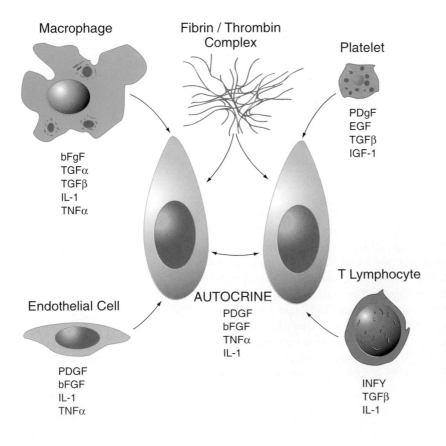

Macrophage

bFgF
TGFα
TGFβ
IL-1
TNFα

Fibrin / Thrombin Complex

Platelet

PDgF
EGF
TGFβ
IGF-1

Endothelial Cell

PDGF
bFGF
IL-1
TNFα

AUTOCRINE
PDGF
bFGF
TNFα
IL-1

T Lymphocyte

INFY
TGFβ
IL-1

Figure 2-24. Control of Smooth Muscle Function. All of the cells within the plaque can produce growth factors modulating smooth muscle cell proliferation and matrix synthesis either in a positive or negative way. bFGF, basic fibroblast growth factor; TGF-αβ, transforming growth factors; IL-1, interleukin-1; TNF-α, tumor necrosis factor-α; EGF, epithelial growth factor; IGF-1, insulin-like growth factor-1; Inf-τ, interferon-τ).

FIBRINOGEN AND PLAQUE EVOLUTION

Fibrinogen-like LDL enters and leaves the intima. Within plaques there is clear evidence of conversion to fibrin (42), which is then degraded via the activity of plasmin. Thrombin is generated locally within the plaque by macrophages and the thrombin/fibrin complex is likely to be a major stimulus of smooth muscle proliferation (Fig. 2-25).

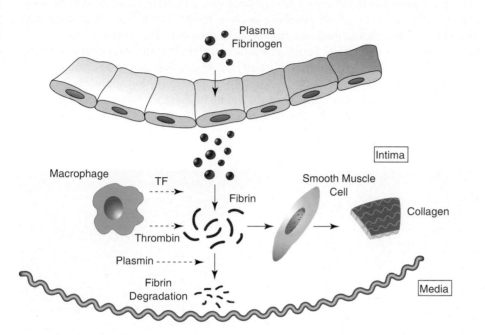
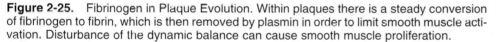

Figure 2-25. Fibrinogen in Plaque Evolution. Within plaques there is a steady conversion of fibrinogen to fibrin, which is then removed by plasmin in order to limit smooth muscle activation. Disturbance of the dynamic balance can cause smooth muscle proliferation.

CALCIFICATION

Plaque calcification is a very common phenomenon (Fig. 2-26). Such calcification occurs in two histological patterns. In one, nodular masses of calcium develop in relation to the lipid core in macrophage-rich areas (Fig. 2-27). More diffuse plate-like areas of calcification (Fig. 2-28) develop in connective tissue in which smooth muscle cells predominate. Calcification is an active and controlled process (43,44) in which both macrophages and smooth muscle cells undergo a phenotypic change and express osteopontin, gelatinase B, bone protein-2, osteocalin, and other features akin to bone-producing cells (45). The whole process closely resembles calcification in bone with the presence of hydroxyapatite and matrix vesicles (46). The nodular masses that develop in the lipid core areas begin as small circular deposits suggesting a matrix vesicle origin. The more diffuse areas of calcification develop as a field change in collagen and may be related to death of smooth muscle cells by apoptosis (47–49). Despite many studies using sophisticated means of visualizing coronary calcification *in vivo*, the degree is a weak predictor of future ischemic events (50) in an individual.

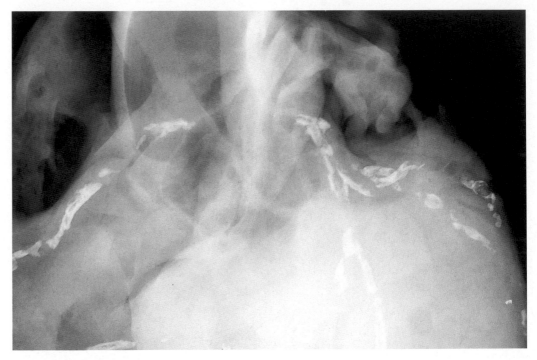

Figure 2-26. Coronary Plaque Calcification. In this x-ray of a heart at necropsy the proximal sections of all three main coronary arteries are outlined by calcification.

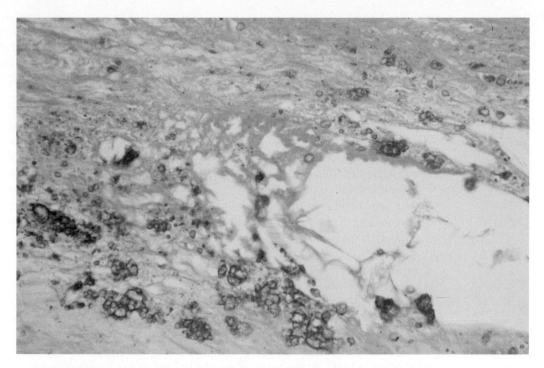

Figure 2-27. Coronary Plaque Calcification. In this section of a plaque adjacent to its lipid core in an area rich in macrophages, calcification is developing as multiple basophilic (*blue-purple*) focal aggregates (hematoxylin and eosin).

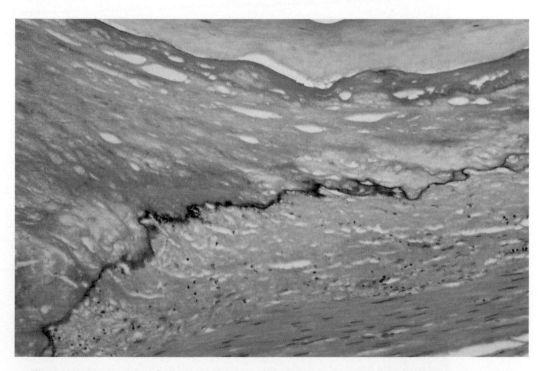

Figure 2-28. Human Coronary Plaque—Calcification. In this histological section of a plaque in the predominantly collagenous areas a wavefront of calcification is seen as a basophilic waving line. This form of calcification produces plates of circumferential-arranged calcified material (hematoxylin and eosin).

ADVENTITIAL INFLAMMATION AND VASCULARIZATION

Viewed externally at surgical operations or at autopsy the adventitia of coronary arteries often appears red, congested, and inflamed. Histological examination confirms that there is a heavy chronic inflammatory infiltrate in the adventitia in which T- and B-lymphocytes, plasma cells, basophils, and macrophages are present. The presence of B-lymphocytes and plasma cells contrasts to the cell population within the intima, where virtually only T-lymphocytes are found. The adventitial response is thought to be an immune reaction to oxidized LDL leaching from the underlying plaque. Oxidized LDL is antigenic and antibodies to it are generated in the adventitia by B-lymphocytes and plasma cells. These antibodies may feed back to form immune complexes with oxidized lipid within the vessel, which are taken up by macrophages, thus enhancing foam cell formation. Immune complexes may play a role in the destruction of the aortic wall in abdominal aortic aneurysms. Circulating levels of antibodies to oxidized LDL may also give an indication of the extent of atherosclerotic disease (51). Along with the adventitial inflammation, vascularity is markedly increased (Figs. 2-29, 2-30). In the normal coronary artery the media is avascular but once intimal plaques form, new vessels begin to penetrate from the adventitia, pass through the media, cross the internal elastic lamina, and enter the base of the plaque (52). These new vessels are sinusoidal rather than clearly arterial, venous, or capillary but have an endothelial lining in which adhesion molecule expression is high (53). Once the plaque is vascularized an alternative entry path for macrophages exists in addition to that coming across the endothelium of the main arterial lumen.

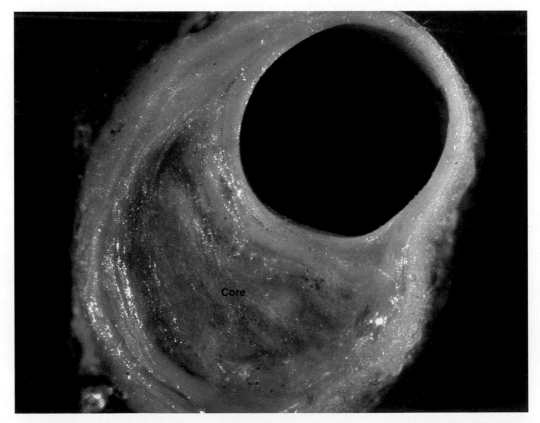

Figure 2-29. Angiographically Invisible Plaque. In this cross section of a large plaque from a segment of artery that was angiographically normal in life, the lumen is round. The plaque is large but bulges entirely outward, giving rise to an eccentric bulge on the outside of the artery. The tissue has been stained with a lipid seeking dye (oil red O) and the core is stained red.

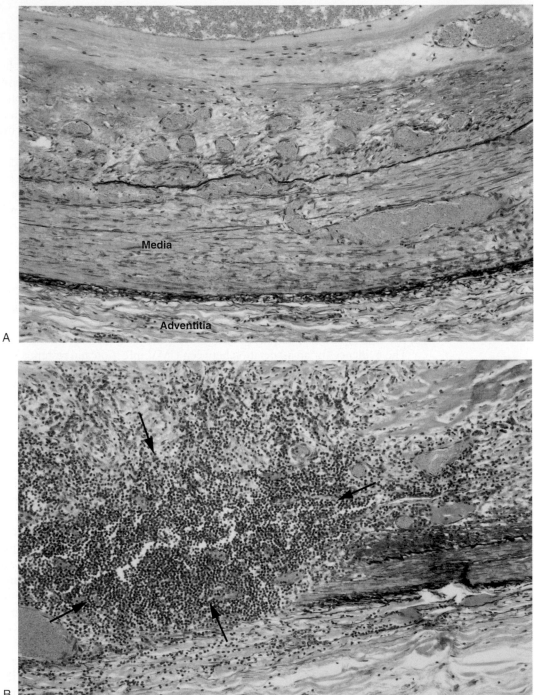

Figure 2-30. Plaque Neovascularization. **A**. Small blood vessels containing contrast media injected at necropsy enter the base of the plaque from the media, which has been vascularized from the adventitia. **B**. In areas of vascularization of the base of the plaque an intense lymphocyte and plasma cell infiltrate (*arrows*) may extend into the media from the adventitia. Such areas are associated with medial destruction and in the aorta may play a role in aneurysm formation.

INFECTIOUS AGENTS AND ATHEROSCLEROSIS

Many years ago it was recognized that avian herpesvirus in chickens can cause an arterial disease with some morphological similarities to atherosclerosis.

A member of this group, cytomegalovirus (CMV), commonly infects humans with frequencies of 50% to 100%, depending on social factors. In immunocompetent individuals, infection is asymptomatic but can be reactivated from a latent phase by other infections or any reduction in immune competence. The virus remains latent in bone marrow cells, endothelial cells, and monocytes; these last two cells having relevance to atherosclerosis, leading to the hypothesis that reactivation of CMV replication might enhance plaque growth. CMV virus certainly has been identified within both two main cell types within human plaques (54). CMV virus can also be found in normal aortic tissue, as well as in plaques in the same individual (55). Evidence for a link between CMV-positive serology indicating carriage of the virus by an individual and the risk of developing symptomatic ischemic heart disease is modest. A study of carotid intimal/medial thickness in the Atherosclerosis Risk in Communities (ARIC) study showed that in 150 subjects with the highest wall thickness when compared to those 150 with the lowest, the levels of CMV titer were different at the $p = 0.013$ level, described as being compatible with a casual link (56). A study of 314 individuals undergoing cardiac transplantation, however, found that CMV-seropositive status was not an independent variable in determining whether there was ischemic heart disease as the cause for transplant (57–59).

The evidence for an association between CMV infection and restenosis is somewhat stronger. In one study (60), in the 49 of 74 patients who were seropositive for CMV the rate of restenosis was higher (43% vs. 8%). An interaction between the immediate early protein IE84 synthesized by the virus soon after reactivation and the p53 tumor-suppressor protein in smooth muscle cells is known to occur and could lead to enhanced smooth muscle proliferation (61).

Chlamydia pneumoniae is a widespread respiratory pathogen and is an obligate intracellular bacterium. Its affinity for living inside monocyte/macrophage cell lines again raises the question of whether it has a potentiating action on atherosclerosis. Repeated subclinical attacks or a chronic infective state are common. Chlamydia organisms have been demonstrated within plaques by polymerase chain reaction (PCR), immunohistochemistry, and culture but not within the normal arterial wall in the same individual (62–64). The organism appears to be present predominantly in macrophages and foam cells (Fig. 2-31), but is also reported by some to occur in smooth muscle cells. Epidemiological studies consistently report a relation between clinically expressed coronary disease and chlamydia seropositivity. In the Helsinki Heart Study, 17% of cases were seropositive for immunoglobulin gamma A (IgA) to chlamydia, compared to 8% of controls (65). The odds ratio of risk of developing clinical symptoms from ischemic heart disease is approximately 2:5 when seropositive and seronegative subjects are compared (65,66). One pilot study reports a beneficial affect on outcomes in unstable angina from an antichlamydial drug (67). In 66 patients treated with roxithromycin, as compared with 63 on placebo, the number who died or had infarction or recurrent angina was 9 versus 2 ($p = 0.064$). The calculated size of a study to confirm a 20% reduction in events by roxithromycin was 3,964 patients. Another pilot study suggested that in subjects with increased levels of antibody to chlamydia, a course of azithromycin may reduce subsequent acute ischemic events in survivors of myocardial infarction (68).

The whole question of the role of chlamydia in relation to atherosclerosis has been recently subjected to metaanalysis (69). The conclusion was that the hypothesis that chlamydia may be causative of atherosclerosis was considered plausible but unproven.

Epidemiological evidence also links *Helicobacter pylori* infection with an increased risk of ischemic heart disease (69). *H. pylori* is a Gram-negative bacteria resident in the upper gastrointestinal tract of up to 60% of subjects over 45 years of age. It induces chronic gastritis and has been causally linked to chronic peptic ulceration and to gastric carcinoma. A number of epidemiological studies have shown an association of *H. pylori*-seropositivity and ischemic heart disease. One study found electrocardiogram (ECG) evidence of chronic ischemic changes to be more common in seropositive individuals by an odds ratio of 3:8, another study put the odds ratio at 1:5 after controlling for social class and other risk factors (70,71). The British Regional Heart Study (72) found that 40- to 59-year-old men developing acute myocardial infarction were more likely to be *H. pylori* seropostive (70% vs. 57%), but after controlling for other risk factors, the odds ratio was only 1:31 for nonfatal and 1:56 for fatal events. There is no current evidence to confirm that *H. pylori* become resident within plaques in a manner analogous to chlamydia.

It seems unlikely that any of these three infections can initiate atherosclerosis on their own, but they probably act as cofactors by enhancing the inflammatory component of atherosclerosis.

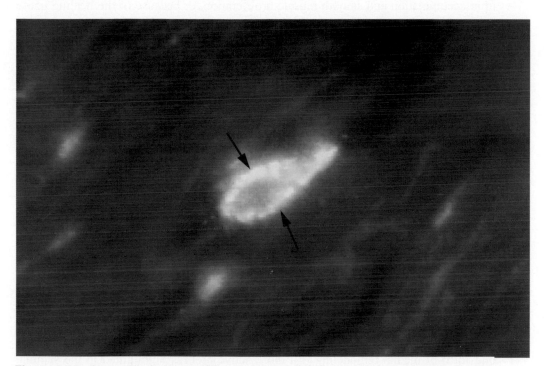

Figure 2-31. Chlamydia in Human Plaque. This section of a human coronary plaque has been treated with a fluorescein-labeled antibody to the polysaccharide capsular antigen common to all the chlamydia species. A macrophage contains several fluorescent bodies (*arrows*) identified by this immunohistochemical technique to be chlamydia organisms.

ATHEROSCLEROSIS AND CLINICAL SYMPTOMS

Coronary disease produces symptoms by a variety of mechanisms. Endothelial function, both in arteries directly affected by atherosclerosis and as a more generalized affect, is abnormal, resulting in a general disturbance in vasomotor tone. The early manifestation is the loss of the normal exercise-induced coronary dilation. Very localized areas of excessive vasoconstriction may develop at the sites of eccentric plaques.

The vast majority of the acute manifestations of coronary disease are the result of thrombus occurring in relation to a plaque leading either to total occlusion or to exposed mural (nonoccluding) thrombus with residual antegrade flow that carries platelet microemboli into the distal vascular bed.

Chronic obstruction to flow occurs when stenosis due to a plaque is sufficiently severe to be flow-limiting on exercise, usually implying at least 50% diameter reduction. Such chronic obstruction either arises because a plaque becomes sufficiently large to encroach on the lumen due to the primary processes of atherogenesis, i.e., lipid accumulation and smooth muscle proliferation, or because of the healing phase of a previous thrombotic event.

Coronary Atherosclerosis, Medial Remodeling, and Ectasia

The practical clinical use of coronary angiography in defining the sites of flow-limiting stenoses and providing data on which interventions are based obscures the fact that angiography is a very insensitive method of detecting plaques. A very large number of plaques go undetected and are hidden in segments of artery that are angiographically normal or, at worst, slightly irregular in outline. This fact was clear for many years from pathology studies but has now been reinforced by intravascular ultrasound (73,74). Even in conditions such as familial hypercholesterolemia plaque-containing arterial segments can be angiographically normal (75).

The insensitivity of angiography is based on two rather different processes, both of which can be termed *medial remodeling*. The term *compensatory dilatation of a coronary artery* is also used and has become widely adopted in intravascular ultrasound studies. The first mechanism is passive. The media behind an eccentric plaque often undergoes atrophy and thins while the media in the uninvolved segment of artery remains normal in structure. The local medial atrophy is associated with loss of smooth muscle cells, the mechanism of which is unclear. The result, however, is that the plaque bulges outward rather than inward (Fig. 2-32). In extreme cases the internal elastic lamina breaks and the plaque is virtually extruded from the artery. The second form of medial remodeling is a more active process highlighted in the seminal work of Glagov and his colleagues (76). As atherosclerosis develops, the vessel wall increases its overall external dimensions to accommodate the plaque while preserving the lumen dimensions. The media and adventitia are now seen as a dynamic tissue rather than as immutable in shape and size. The factors and signaling mechanisms that locally control remodeling must involve both degradation and synthesis of connective tissue matrix with smooth muscle cell, movement and rearrangement have not been studied in detail.

The development of coronary stenosis can therefore be seen as a change in the balance between the plaque growing and the vessel wall undergoing compensatory remodeling (77,78). In some patients, compensatory dilatation seems to be minimal, in others it is a major factor in preventing stenosis. Even within individual patients some segments of artery remodel while others do not. The role of compensatory dilatation in the development of stenosis is discussed in Chapter 4.

Ectasia (Figs. 2-32, 2-33) is related to medial remodeling in that a segment of artery undergoes a marked increase in diameter, as compared with adjacent segments of normal artery. The phenomenon is age-related and associated with diffuse medial atrophy and loss of smooth muscle cells. There is usually diffuse intimal involvement by atherosclerosis without discrete plaque formation.

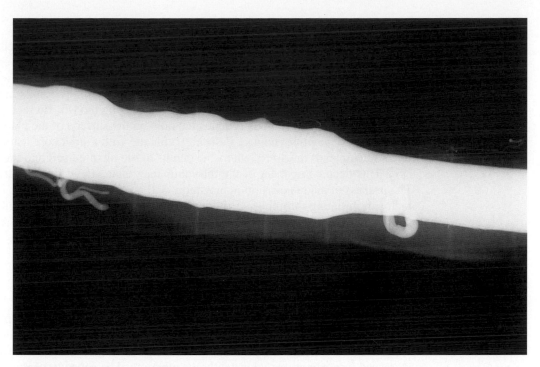

Figure 2-32. Coronary Ectasia. In one segment of right coronary artery there is an irregular outline indicating plaques are present. The diameter of the artery is, however, larger than the smooth segment of normal coronary artery.

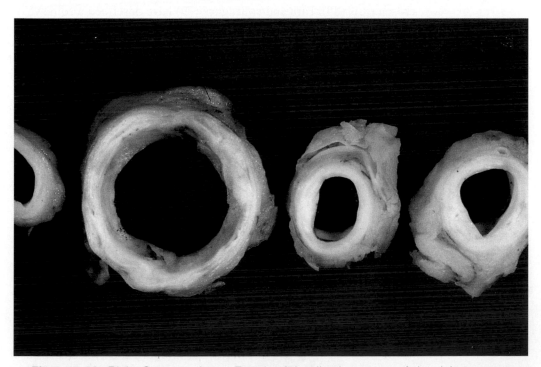

Figure 2-33. Right Coronary Artery Ectasia. A localized segment of the right coronary artery has dilated to approximately three times the normal diameter shown in proximal and distal portions of the artery.

MECHANISMS OF THROMBOSIS AND ATHEROSCLEROSIS

Thrombosis in relation to plaques occurs because of two separate mechanisms (Fig. 2-34). In endothelial erosion (denudation), the endothelial covering over a plaque is lost, exposing collagen, Von Willebrand Factor, and fibronectin, and leading to adhesion of a monolayer of platelets over the area (79,80). This thrombus may then grow by the aggregation and adhesion of more platelets using the IIb/IIIa receptor and binding fibrinogen. The thrombus is deposited only on the surface of the plaque. In plaque disruption (synonyms: rupture, fissuring) a plaque with a lipid core tears open. Blood from the lumen of the artery enters the depths of the plaque itself and thrombus forms (81). This deep component of the thrombus may then extend into the arterial lumen. The process of plaque disruption inevitably will involve endothelial loss, but the major factor in initiating thrombosis is contact of blood with the highly thrombogenic lipid core. The other essential difference between endothelial erosion and disruption is that the former has thrombus on the plaque surface while in the latter there is a component within the plaque in addition to that in the lumen.

Endothelial Erosion

Minor degrees of endothelial denudation consistently develop once plaque formation is established (34,35) (Fig. 2-35). This fact has two important functional implications. First, it must indicate that the endothelial cells in atherosclerotic arteries have an increased turnover and are constantly regenerating. The capacity of regenerating cells to produce nitric oxides is reduced. Second, platelet-derived growth factors that can influence smooth muscle proliferation are being produced. Endothelial erosion is seen over plaques once significant macrophage foam cell densities occur in the superficial zones of the intima and is usually regarded as part of the inflammatory process in atherosclerosis (80). Farb and colleagues (79) have described a somewhat different form of endothelial erosion unrelated to macrophage activity. In young women, they describe thrombus occurring on the surface of plaques without a lipid component and with predominantly a smooth muscle and proteoglycan composition. Larger areas of endothelial denudation can lead to larger thrombi (Fig. 2-36), which can become occlusive (Fig. 2-37).

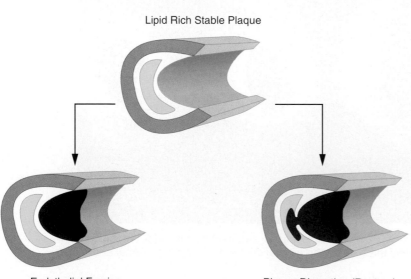

Lipid Rich Stable Plaque

Endothelial Erosion

Plaque Disruption (Rupture)

Figure 2-34. Mechanisms of Thrombus in Atherosclerosis. In endothelial erosion the thrombus is superficial, i.e., on the surface of the plaque. In disruption there is a component deep in the plaque and a component in the lumen.

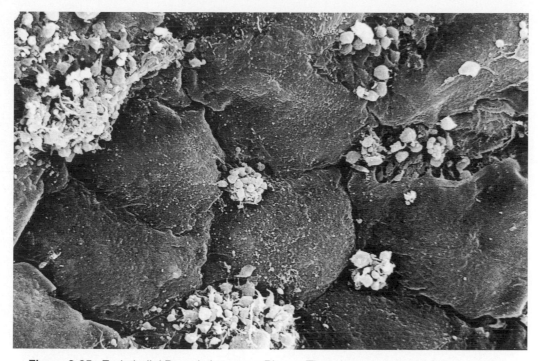

Figure 2-35. Endothelial Denudation over a Plaque. There is an area in which the endothelium has been lost, although the adjacent endothelial cells appear intact. Some platelets adhere to the exposed subendothelial matrix. Scanning electron microscopy.

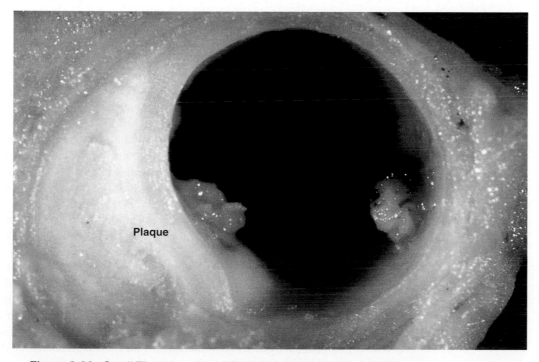

Plaque

Figure 2-36. Small Thrombus due to Endothelial Erosion. Two small thrombi approximately 1.5 mm in diameter adherent to the endothelial surface of a plaque, which is intact and shows no disruption.

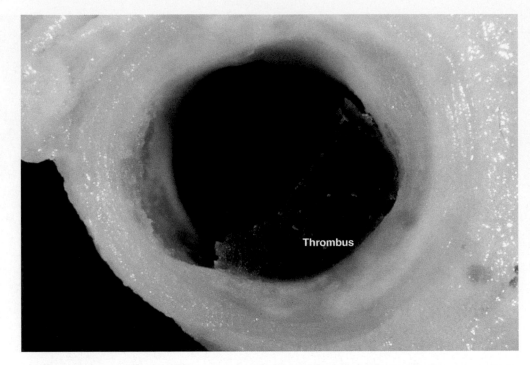

Figure 2-37. Large Thrombus due to Endothelial Erosion. A thrombus large enough to influence flow and be visible on angiography is adherent to the endothelial surface of an intact plaque.

Plaque Disruption: The Vulnerable Plaque

Disruption (Fig. 2-38) is a complication of plaques with certain well-defined characteristics. These characteristics include a lipid core that occupies over 40% of plaque volume, a lipid core without a supporting internal collagen matrix, a thin plaque cap, a high density of macrophages, and a reduced density of smooth cells in the cap (82,83). Concordance of these characteristics define what has become known as a vulnerable plaque—that is, it has a high risk of a future disruption episode. Plaque vulnerability is not an absolute but a relative quality of plaques. Lipid cores and macrophage infiltration are present in the great majority of plaques; high vulnerability occurs when all the factors coincide in a particular plaque (84). Vulnerable plaques are distributed across the whole range of plaque size and the degree of stenosis. This has the implication that angiography cannot give any indication of the site and frequency of vulnerable plaques in the coronary arteries (85). The fact that highly vulnerable plaques are often either angiographically invisible or cause minor stenosis is the explanation for the fact that thrombi causing infarction develop in such arterial segments. After thrombolysis the residual stenosis may not be severe (86).

The properties of the cap tissue plays a major part in resistance to plaque disruption. The mechanical strength of the cap is dependent on both the amount of collagen and the spatial organization of the collagen fibrils and its proteoglycan matrix. This matrix is produced and maintained by smooth muscle cells that lie in lacunae in the cap tissue. Cap tears are due to combinations of an increased mechanical load placed on the tissue and a reduction in the innate mechanical strength of the cap itself. The increased mechanical load imposed on plaque caps has been largely studied by computer simulation of events in systole in plaques using finite element analysis (87,88). Such computer modeling shows that plaques with a large lipid core and a thin cap, particularly if they do not cause stenosis, are mechanically inefficient. Circumferential wall stress in systole is normally evenly distributed across the artery wall; a plaque core that is soft cannot carry this load, which therefore has to be redistributed. The redistribution throws most of the stress onto the cap tissue with focal point concentrations up to ten times the normal. The insertion of the cap into the more normal vessel wall, a common site of cap tears, often has the highest stress.

The aspect of the innate strength of cap tissue has largely been studied by mechanical testing *in vitro* of samples obtained at autopsy or surgery (89). Such studies show that the amount of collagen, its organization and proteoglycan concentrations are the determinants of strength.

Plaque caps are being increasingly seen as dynamic structures in which the collagen synthesis by smooth muscle cells is balanced by degradation of matrix by metalloproteinases (Fig. 2-39). The balance determines cap strength and if the balance is tipped to degradation mediated by macrophages and basophils in an inflammatory process, the cap weakens. The tissue degradation is often very focal and if this coincides with a focal area of high stress on the cap, ruptures occurs.

The production of collagen and other matrix products by smooth muscle cells is modulated by a number of factors, but may be inhibited by interferon-τ produced by T-lymphocytes within the plaque (90). The fall in smooth muscle cell numbers in plaque caps is likely to be due to apoptosis and there is evidence that this is triggered by proximity to macrophages (49). A range of enzymes capable of reducing collagen to low molecular weight fragments and thus destroying the cap tissue are present in plaques. The best characterized are the metalloproteinase family individual members, which can destroy any of the connective tissue components (29). Members of this family are secreted in an inactive form and activated by plasmin in the tissue. Tissue inhibitors of these proteinases (TIMPs) are also produced and whether focal destruction of matrix occurs depends on the relative amounts of enzyme and inhibitor. Work on human plaques shows both the presence of the enzymes (91) and that they are active in destroying matrix (92). The predominant cell producing metalloproteinases is likely to be the macrophage, but most cells also produce similar enzymes and can also initiate activation of metalloproteinases without plasmin. Mast-cell accumulation at the site of plaque tears has been reported (93). Mast cells can also produce tumor necrosis factor-α (TNF-α), a potent initiator of macrophage secretion of metalloproteinases (94).

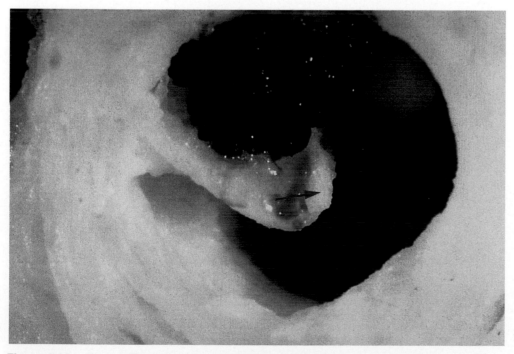

Figure 2-38. Plaque Disruption. A plaque cap has torn and projects upward (*arrow*) into the coronary artery lumen. The bed of the exposed lipid core is filled with thrombus.

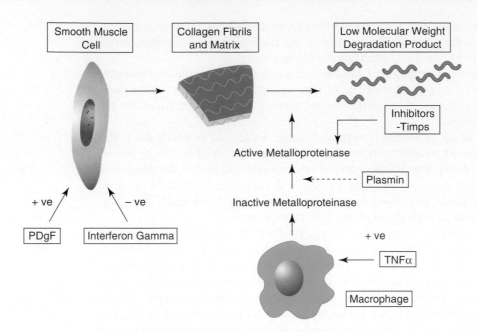

Figure 2-39. Plaque Cap Dynamics. The mechanical strength of the cap depends on collagen produced by smooth muscle cells. Some factors [e.g., platelet-derived growth factor (PDGF)] will stimulate collagen synthesis—others, such as interferon-γ inhibit it. Metalloproteinases produced by macrophages and perhaps basophils degrade the collagen.

REFERENCES

1. Ross R. The pathogenesis of atherosclerosis—a perspective for the 1990s. *Nature* 1993;362:801–809.
2. Stary H, Chandler A, Dinsmore R, et al. A definition of advanced types of atherosclerotic lesions and a histological classification of atherosclerosis. A report from the Committee on vascular lesions of the Council on Atherosclerosis, American Heart Association. *Circulation* 1995;92:1355–1374.
3. Stary HC. Evolution and progression of atherosclerotic lesions in coronary arteries of children and young adults. *Arteriosclerosis* 1989;9:1–19.
4. Wissler, RW. An overview of the quantitative influence of several risk factors on progression of atherosclerosis in young people in the United States. *Am J Med Sci* 1995;310:S29–S36.
5. Strong J. Atherosclerotic lesions. Natural history, risk factors and topography. *Arch Pathol Lab Med* 1992;116:1268–1275.
6. PDAY RG. Natural history of aortic and coronary atherosclerotic lesions in youth: findings from the PDAY study. *Arterioscler Thromb Vasc Biol* 1993;13:1291–1298.
7. Tracy RE, Newman WP, Wattigney WA, et al. Risk factors and atherosclerosis in young: autopsy findings of the Bogalusa Heart Study. *Am J Med Sci* 1995;310:S37–S41.
8. McGill HC. *The geographic pathology of atherosclerosis.* Baltimore: Williams & Wilkins, 1968:453–465.
9. Faggiotto A, Ross R, Harker L. Studies of hypercholesterolaemia in the non-human primate: I. Changes that lead to fatty streak formation. *Arteriosclerosis* 1984;4:323–340.
10. Steinberg D, Witztum JL. Lipoproteins and atherogenesis. *JAMA* 1990;264:3047–3052.
11. Berliner JA, Territo MC, Sevanian A, et al. Minimally modified low density lipoprotein stimulates monocyte endothelial interactions. *J Clin Invest* 1990;85:1260–1266.
12. Brown M, Goldstein J. Lipoprotein metabolism in the macrophage: implications for cholesterol deposition in atherosclerosis. *Ann Rev Biochem* 1983;52:223–261.
13. Krieger M, Hertz H. Structures and functions of multiligand lipoprotein receptors: macrophage scavenger receptors and LDL receptor-related protein (LRP). *Ann Rev Biochem* 1994;63:601–637.
14. Pearson A. Scavenger receptors in innate immunity. *Curr Opin Immunol* 1996;8:20–28.
15. Suzuki H, Gordon S, Kodama T. Resistance to atherosclerosis and susceptibility to infection in scavenger receptor knockout mice. *Nature* 1997;386:292–296.
16. O'Brien K, Allen M, McDonald T, et al. Vascular cell adhesion molecule-1 is expressed in human coronary atherosclerotic plaques. Implications for the mode of progression of advanced coronary atherosclerosis. *J Clin Invest* 1993;92:945–951.
17. de Villiers W, Fraser I, Hughes D, Doyle A, Gordon S. Macrophage-colony-stimulating factor selectively enhances macrophage scavenger receptor expression and function. *J Exp Med* 1994;180:705–709.
18. Nelken NA, Coughlin SR, Gordon D, Wilcox JN. Monocyte chemoattractant protein-1 in human atheromatous plaques. *J Clin Invest* 1993;92:1121–1127.
19. Rosenfeld ME, Yla-Herttuala S, Lipton BA, et al. Macrophage colony-stimulation factor mRNA and protein in atherosclerotic lesions of rabbits and man. *Am J Pathol* 1992;140:291–300.
20. Yla-Herttuala S, Palinski W, Rosenfeld ME, et al. Evidence for the presence of oxidatively modified low density lipoprotein in atherosclerotic lesions of rabbit and man. *J Clin Invest* 1989;84:1086–1095.
21. Mitchinson M, Hothersall D, Brooks P, De Burbure C. The distribution of ceroid in human atherosclerosis. *J Pathol* 1985;145:177–183.
22. Toschi V, Gallo R, Lettino M, et al. Tissue factor modulates the thrombogenicity of human atherosclerotic plaques. *Circulation* 1997;95:594–599.
23. Marmur JD, Thiruvikraman SV, Fyfe BS, et al. Identification of active Tissue Factor in human coronary atheroma. *Circulation* 1996;94:1226–1232.
24. Mach F, Schonbeck U, Bonnefoy J-Y et al. Activation of monocyte/macrophage functions related to acute atheroma complication by ligation of CD-40. *Circulation* 1997;96:396–399.
25. Guyton J, Klemp K. Development of the atherosclerotic core region: chemical and ultrastructural analysis of microdissected atherosclerotic lesions from human aorta. *Arterioscler Thromb Vasc Biol* 1994;14:1305–1314.
26. Hegyl L, Skepper J, Cary N, Mitchinson M. Foam cell apoptosis and the development of the lipid core of human atherosclerosis. *J Pathol* 1996;179:249–302.
27. Geng Y, Libby P. Evidence for apoptosis in advanced human atheroma. Colocalization with interleukin-1 beta-converting enzyme. *Am J Pathol* 1995;147:151–266.
28. Mitchinson M, Hardwick S, Bennett M. Cell death in atherosclerotic plaques. *Curr Opin Lipidol* 1996;7:324–329.
29. Dollery CM, Mcewan JR, Henney A. Matrix metalloproteinases and cardiovascular disease. *Circ Res* 1995;77:863–868.
30. Zeiher A, Drexler H, Wollschlager H, Just H. Modulation of coronary vasomotor tone in humans: progressive endothelial dysfunction with different early stages of coronary atherosclerosis. *Circulation* 1991;83:391–401.
31. Reddy K, Nair R, Sheehan H, Hodgson J. Evidence that selective endothelial dysfunction may occur in the absence of angiographic or ultrasound atherosclerosis in patients with risk factors for atherosclerosis. *J Am Coll Cardiol* 1994;23:833–843.
32. Celermajer D, Sorensen K, Bull C, Robinson J, Deanfield J. Endothelium-dependent dilation in the systemic arteries of asymptomatic subjects relates to coronary risk factors and their interaction. *J Am Coll Cardiol* 1994;24:1468–1474.
33. Deckert V, Persegol L, Viens L, et al. Inhibitors of arterial relaxation among components of human oxidized low-density lipoproteins. Cholesterol derivatives oxidized in position 7 are potent inhibitors of endothelium-dependent relaxation. *Circulation* 1997;95:723–731.
34. Davies M, Woolf N, Rowles P, Pepper J. Morphology of the endothelium over atherosclerotic plaques in human coronary arteries. *Br Heart J* 1988;60:459–464.
35. Burrig K. The endothelium of advanced arteriosclerotic plaques in humans. *Arterioscler Thromb Vasc Biol* 1991;11:1678–1689.

36. Stary H, Blankenhorn D, Chandler A, Glagov S. A definition of the intima of human arteries and of its atherosclerosis-prone regions: a report from the Committee on Vascular Lesions of the Council on Arteriosclerosis, American Heart Associations, Special Report. *Circulation* 1992;85:391–405.

37. Raines EW, Ross R. Smooth muscle cells and the pathogenesis of the lesions of atherosclerosis. *Br Heart J* 1993;69:S30–S37.

38. Hart C, Clowes A. Platelet-derived growth factor and arterial response to injury. *Circulation* 1997;95: 555–556.

39. Sirois MG, Simons M, Edelman ER. Antisense oligonucleotide inhibition of PDGFR-beta receptor subunit expression directs suppression of intimal thickening. *Circulation* 1997;65:669–676.

40. Medalion B, Merin G, Aingorn H, et al. Endogenous basic fibroblast growth factor displaced by heparin from the lumenal surface of human blood vessels is preferentially sequestered by injured regions of the vessel wall. *Circulation* 1997;95:1853–1862.

41. Lindner V, Reidy M. Proliferation of smooth muscle cells after vascular injury is inhibited by an antibody against basic fibroblast growth factor. *Proc Natl Acad Sci USA* 1991;88:3739–3743.

42. Bini A, Fenoglio J, Mesa-Tejada R, Kudryk B, Kaplan K. Identification and distribution of fibrinogen, fibrin and fibrin(ogen) degradation products in atherosclerosis. Use of monoclonal antibodies. *Arteriosclerosis* 1989;9:109–121.

43. Balica M, Bostrom K, Shin V, Tillisch K, Demer L. Calcifying subpopulation of bovine aortic smooth muscle cells is responsive to 17B-estradiol. *Circulation* 1997;95:1954–1960.

44. Giachelli C, Bae N, Almeida M, Denhardt D, CE A, Schwartz S. Osteopontin is elevated during neointima formation in rat arteries and is a novel component of human atherosclerotic plaques. *J Clin Invest* 1993;92:1686–1696.

45. Shanahan C, Weissberg P, Metcalfe J. Isolation of gene markers of differentiated and proliferating vascular smooth muscle cells. *Circ Res* 1993;73:193–204.

46. Kim K. Calcification of matrix vesicles in human aortic valve and aortic media. *Fed Proc* 1976;35:156–162.

47. Kockx M, De Meyer G, Muhring J, Bult H, Bultinck J, Herman A. Distribution of cell replication and apoptosis in atherosclerotic plaques of cholesterol-fed rabbits. *Atherosclerosis* 1996;120:115–124.

48. Kockx M, De Meyer G. Apoptosis in human atherosclerosis and restenosis. *Circulation* 1996;93:394–395.

49. Kockx MM, de Meyer GRY, Bortier H, et al. Luminal foam cell accumulation is associated with smooth muscle cell death in the intimal thickening of human saphenous vein grafts. *Circulation* 1996;94:1255–1262.

50. Secci A, Wong N, Tang W, et al. Electron beam computed tomographic coronary calcium as a predictor of coronary events. Comparison of two protocols. *Circulation* 1997;96:1122–1129.

51. Salonen J, Yla-Herttuala S, Yamamoto R, et al. Auto-antibody against oxidised LDL and progression of carotid atherosclerosis. *Lancet* 1992;339:883–887.

52. Barger A, Beeuwkes R, Lainey L, Silverman K. Hypothesis: vaso vasorum and neovascularization of human coronary arteries: a possible role in the pathophysiology of atherosclerosis. *N Engl J Med* 1984;310:175–177.

53. O'Brien K, McDonald T, Chait A, Allen M, Alpers C. Neovascular expression of E-selectin, intercellular adhesion molecule-1, and vascular cell adhesion molecule-1 in human atherosclerosis and their relation to intimal leukocyte content. *Circulation* 1996;93:672–682.

54. Kuo C, Gown A, Benditt E, Grayston J. Detection of *Chlamydia pneumoniae* in aortic lesions of atherosclerosis by immunocytochemical stain. *Arterioscler Thromb Vasc Biol* 1993;13:1501–1504.

55. Melnick J, Hu C, Burek J, Adam E, DeBakey M. Cytomegalovirus DNA in arterial walls of patients with atherosclerosis. *J Med Virol* 1994;42:170–174.

56. Nieto F, Adam E, Sorlie P, et al. Cohort study of cytomegalovirus infection as a risk factor for carotid intimal-medial thickening, a measure of subclinical atherosclerosis. *Circulation* 1996;94:922–927.

57. Fernando S, Booth J, Boriskin Y et al. Association of cytomegalovirus infection with post-transplantation cardiac rejection as studied using the polymerase chain rection. *J Med Virol* 1994;42:396–404.

58. Lowry RW, Adam E, Hu C, et al. What are the implications of cardiac infection with cytomegalovirus before heart transplantation. *J Heart Lung Transplant* 1994;13:122–128.

59. Dummer S, Lee A, Breinig MK, Kormos R, et al. Investigation of cytomegalovirus infection as a risk factor for coronary atherosclerosis in the explanted hearts for patients undergoing heart transplantation. *J Med Virol* 1994;44:305–309.

60. Zhou Y, Leon M, Waclawiw M, et al. Association between prior cytomegalovirus infection and the risk of restenosis after coronary atherectomy. *N Engl J Med* 1996;335:624–630.

61. Speir E, Modali R, Huang E, et al. Potential role of human cytomegalovirus and p53 interaction in coronary restenosis. *Science* 1994;265:391–394.

62. Kuo C, Grayston J, Campbell L. *Chlamydia pneumoniae* (TWAR) in coronary arteries of young adults (15–34 years old). *Proc Natl Acad Sci USA* 1995;92:6911–6914.

63. Grayston J, Kuo C, Coulson A. *Chlamydia pneumoniae* (TWAR) in atherosclerosis of the carotid artery. *Circulation* 1995;92:3397–3400.

64. Muhlestein JB, Hammond EH, Carlquist JF, et al. Increased incidence of chlamydia species within the coronary arteries of patients with symptomatic atherosclerotic versus other forms of cardiovascular disease. *J Am Coll Cardiol* 1996;27:1555–1556.

65. Saikku P, Leiononen M, Tenkanen L. Chronic *Chlamydia pneumoniae* infection as a risk factor for coronary heart disease in the Helsinki Heart Study. *Ann Intern Med* 1992;116:273–277.

66. Saikku P, Mattila K, Nieminen M. Serological evidence of an association of a novel chlamydia, TWAR, with chronic coronary heart disease and acute myocardial infarction. *Lancet* 1988;ii:983–986.

67. Gurfinkel E, Bozovich G, Daroca A, Beck E, Mautner B for the ROXIS Study Group. Randomised trial of roxithromycin in non-Q wave coronary syndromes: ROXIS pilot study. *Lancet* 1997;350:404–407.

68. Gupta S, Leatham EW, Carrington D, et al. Elevated *Chlamydia pneumoniae* antibodies, cardiovascular events and azithromycin in male survivors of myocardial infarction. *Circulation* 1997;96:404–407.

69. Danesh J, Collins R, Peto R. Chronic infections and coronary heart disease: Is there a link? *Lancet* 1997;350:430–436.

70. Patel P, Mendall M, Stephens J. Association of *Helicobacter pylori* and *Chlamydia pneumoniae* infections with coronary heart disease and cardiovascular risk factors. *Br Med J* 1995;311:711–714.
71. Murray L, Bamford K, O'Reilly D. *Helicobacter pylori* infection: relationship with cardiovascular risk factors, ischaemic heart disease, and social class. *Br Heart J* 1995;74:497–501.
72. Whincup P, Mendall M, Perry I. Prospective relationships between *Helicobacter pylori* infection, coronary heart disease and stroke in middle aged men. *Heart* 1996;75:568– 572.
73. Mintz G, Painter J, Pichard A, et al. Atherosclerosis in angiographically "normal" coronary artery reference segments: an intravascular ultrasound study with clinical correlations. *J Am Coll Cardiol* 1995;25: 1479–1485.
74. Tuzcu E, Hobbs R, Rincon G, et al. Occult and frequent transmission of atherosclerotic coronary disease with cardiac transplantation. Insights from intravascular ultrasound. *Circulation* 1995;91:1706–1713.
75. Hausmann D, Johnsoin JA, Sudhir K, et al. Angiographically silent atherosclerosis detected by intravascular ultrasound in patients with familial hypercholesterolemia and familial combined hyperlipidemia: correlation with high density lipoproteins. *J Am Coll Cardiol* 1996;27:1562–1570.
76. Glagov S, Weisenberd E, Zarins C, Stankunavicius R, Kolettis G. Compensatory enlargement of human atherosclerotic coronary arteries. *N Engl J Med* 1987;316:1371–1375.
77. Nishioka T, Luo H, Eigler N, Berglund H, Kim C-J, Siegel R. Contribution of inadequate compensatory enlargement to development of human coronary artery stenosis: an in vivo intravascular ultrasound study. *J Am Coll Cardiol* 1996;27:1571–1576.
78. Mintz G, Kent K, Pichard A, Satler L, Popma J, Leon M. Contribution of inadequate arterial remodeling to the development of focal coronary artery stenoses. An intravascular ultrasound study. *Circulation* 1997;95: 1791–1798.
79. Farb A, Burke A, Tang A, et al. Coronary plaque erosion without rupture into a lipid core. A frequent cause of coronary thrombosis in sudden coronary death. *Circulation* 1996;93:1354–1363.
80. van der Wal A, Becker A, van der Loos C, Das P. Site of intimal rupture or erosion of thrombosed coronary atherosclerotic plaques is characterized by an inflammatory process irrespective of the dominant plaque morphology. *Circulation* 1994;89:36–44.
81. Davies M, Thomas A. Plaque fissuring—the cause of acute myocardial infarction, sudden ischaemic death and crescendo angina. *Br Heart J* 1985;53:363–373.
82. Falk E. Morphological features of unstable atherothrombotic plaques underlying acute coronary syndromes. *Am J Cardiol* 1989;63:114E–120E.
83. Davies M, Richardson P, Woolf N, Katz D, Mann J. Risk of thrombosis in human atherosclerotic plaques: role of extracellular lipid, macrophage, and smooth muscle cell content. *Br Heart J* 1993;69:377–381.
84. Davies M. Stability and instability: two faces of coronary atherosclerosis: The Paul Dudley White lecture 1995. *Circulation* 1996;94:2013–2020.
85. Mann J, Davies M. Vulnerable plaque: relation of characteristics to degree of stenosis in human coronary arteries. *Circulation* 1996;94:928–931.
86. Marshall JC, Waxman HL, Sauerwein A, et al. Frequency of low-grade residual coronary stenosis after thrombolysis during acute myocardial infarction. *Am J Cardiol* 1990;66:773–778.
87. Richardson P, Davies M, Born G. Influence of plaque configuration and stress distribution on fissuring of coronary atherosclerotic plaques. *Lancet* 1989;2:941–944.
88. Cheng G, Loree H, Kamm R, Fishbein M, Lee R. Distribution of circumferential stress in ruptured and stable atherosclerotic lesions. A structural analysis with histopathological correlation. *Circulation* 1993;87: 1179–1187.
89. Lendon C, Davies M, Born G, Richardson P. Atherosclerotic plaque caps are locally weakened when macrophages density is increased. *Atherosclerosis* 1991;87:87–90.
90. Libby P. Molecular bases of the acute coronary syndromes. *Circulation* 1995;91:2844–2850.
91. Henney A, Wakeley P, Davies M, et al. Localization of stromelysin gene expression in atherosclerotic plaques by in situ hybridization. *Proc Natl Acad Sci USA* 1991;88:8154– 8158.
92. Galis Z, Sukhova G, Lark M, Libby P. Increased expression of matrix metalloproteinases and matrix degrading activity in vulnerable regions of human atherosclerotic plaques. *J Clin Invest* 1994;94:2493–2503.
93. Kovanen P, Kaartinen M, Paavonen T. Infiltrates of activated mast cells at the site of coronary atheromatous erosion or rupture in myocardial infarction. *Circulation* 1995;92:1084–1088.
94. Kaartinen M, Penttila A, Kovanen P. Mast cells in rupture-prone areas of human coronary atheromas produce and store TNF-α. *Circulation* 1996;94:2787–2792.

3

The Acute Ischemic Syndromes and Coronary Disease Progression

INTRODUCTION

The clinical spectrum that runs from mild through more severe rest pain to crescendo unstable angina and then to acute regional myocardial infarction is predominantly caused by coronary thrombosis occurring on a culprit atheromatous plaque. This view was firmly established for acute regional infarction by the classic clinical angiographic work of DeWood et al. (1) and Stadius et al. (2) who showed that soon after the onset of infarction the artery subtending the infarct zone was occluded. Subsequently the artery often reopened spontaneously, but this was markedly accelerated by fibrinolytic therapy, emphasizing the role of thrombosis in causing occlusion. In patients who die of acute myocardial infarction in the hospital, particularly if fibrinolysis has not been used therapeutically, it is characteristic in necropsy angiograms to find the artery totally occluded (Figs. 3-1, 3-2). Persistent acute occlusion by thrombosis appears to be a significant factor associated with death, hence its high prevalence in pathology studies (3). In a proportion of patients with regional infarcts, however, there has been reestablishment of antegrade blood flow in the supplying artery, even after the onset of infarction this appears to have long-term benefit (4). The residual angiographic appearances after flow has been reestablished by natural or therapeutic lysis vary widely and give some indication of the degree of plaque distortion and expansion that has occurred following disruption (Figs. 3-3–3-6). Perhaps the most important change in thinking for both clinicians and pathologists in the 1980s was that coronary thrombi were labile dynamic structures. The role of thrombosis in unstable angina was also established by angiographic studies in life. In unstable angina a characteristic form of stenosis was described in which the lesion was eccentric, had irregular outlines with an overhanging edge, and, in a proportion of cases, there was an associated intraluminal filling defect (5). These appearances were designated as type II lesions to distinguish them from stenoses with smooth outlines responsible for stable exertional angina (type I). The classic angiographic/morphological/pathology studies of Levin and Fallon (6) showed that type II lesions were plaques undergoing thrombosis due to disruption. Pathology studies also showed that identical angiographic appearances and episodes of plaque disruption were found in a high proportion of sudden ischemic deaths (7,8).

The dominant role of thrombosis in the acute ischemic syndromes must not, however, prevent the recognition that arterial spasm plays a role and, in an occasional individual patient, may be the main mechanism.

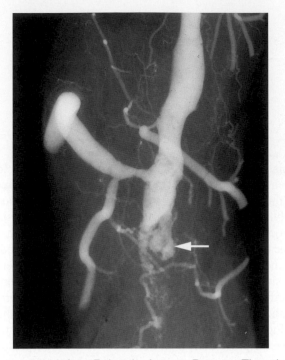

Figure 3-1. Infarct-Related Artery—Recent Thrombotic Occlusion. The vessel comes to an abrupt end with no distal filling. The proximal face of the occlusion (*arrow*) is irregular and lobulated where angiographic media outlines thrombus.

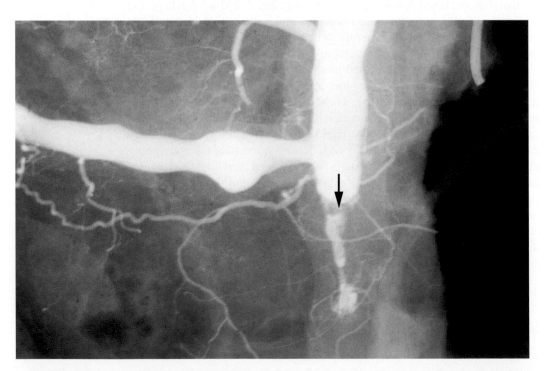

Figure 3-2. Infarct-Related Artery—Recent Total Thrombotic Occlusion. The occluded artery (*arrow*) shows a thread of angiographic medium passing some way into the thrombus but there is no distal artery filling.

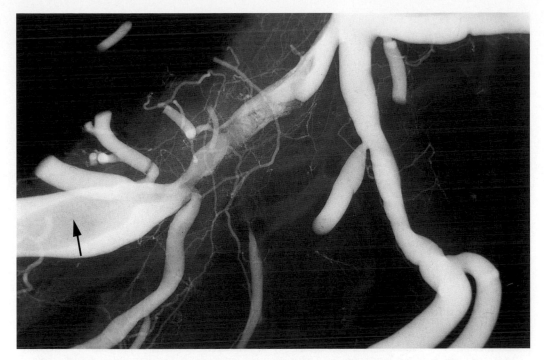

Figure 3-3. Infarct-Related Artery—Recent Thrombus. In this artery there is filling by antegrade flow of an ectatic distal segment of artery. There is a long irregular stenosis with intraluminal thrombus that has a distal tail seen as a filling defect (*arrow*). These angiographic appearances suggest a major disruption of a plaque.

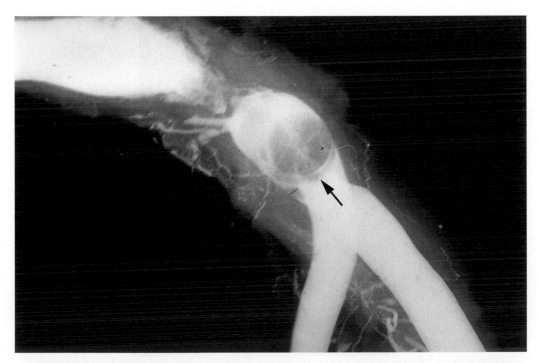

Figure 3-4. Infarct-Related Artery—Recent Thrombus. There is a proximal very high-grade but localized stenosis with a large mass of distal thrombus (*arrow*) within the lumen, but antegrade flow is present. The lesion is due to major but localized disruption of a plaque.

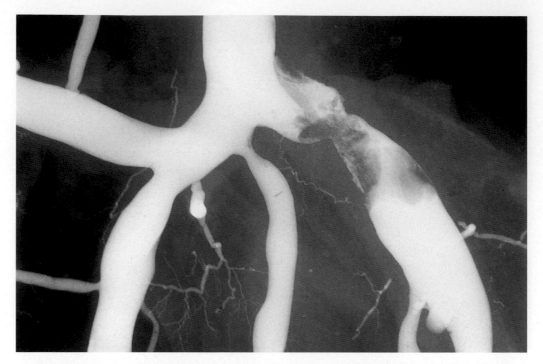

Figure 3-5. Infarct-Related Artery—Recent Thrombus. The left anterior descending coronary artery shows a nonoccluding thrombus attached to a plaque that is causing localized high-grade stenosis but appears dome-shaped and relatively smooth. A major intraplaque component of thrombus was present.

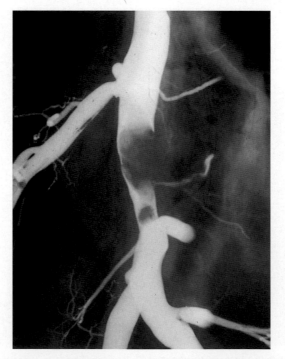

Figure 3-6. Infarct-Related Artery—Recent Thrombus. There is a large intraluminal thrombus but no apparent stenosis or related wall disease. The plaque disruption was minor in a small plaque without an intraplaque thrombotic component and, had the thrombus been lysed and the patient survived, a near normal angiogram may have resulted. The patient appears to have had an exaggerated thrombotic response to a minor plaque event.

ACUTE MYOCARDIAL INFARCTION

The causal role of thrombosis had been emphasized by the majority of pathologists studying acute regional infarction throughout this century (9). One of the most telling studies was a joint clinical pathological approach by Fulton (10). Radiolabeled fibrinogen was given to patients as soon as possible after they developed pain and electrocardiogram (ECG) changes. In those who came to autopsy, the artery supplying the infarction was examined in great detail by autoradiography. This showed that part of the thrombus was radionegative, i.e., predated the injection of the label but the distal part of the thrombus was labeled. This showed convincingly that thrombosis preceded and beyond reasonable doubt caused the infarct, but that thrombus continued to propagate down the artery after the infarct had developed. Similar work was carried out with radiolabeled platelets (11). The challenge then became to understand what event precipitated thrombosis over a particular plaque at that particular point in time. As emphasized in Chapter 2, two processes, plaque disruption (rupture) and endothelial erosion, are responsible. There is a wide spectrum in the appearances of plaque-rupture–related thrombi causing acute myocardial infarction. In some there is preexisting high-grade stenosis and the thrombus is largely within the lumen with a fissure leading down into the lipid core (Fig. 3-7). In other plaques, both those causing significant prior stenosis and those with less degree of prior stenosis, the intraluminal and intraplaque components of the thrombus are more equal in size (Figs. 3-8, 3-9). Finally, some plaques are disrupted to a degree that it is impossible to determine prior plaque size and the lumen is occluded by a mixture of plaque debris and thrombus (Fig. 3-10).

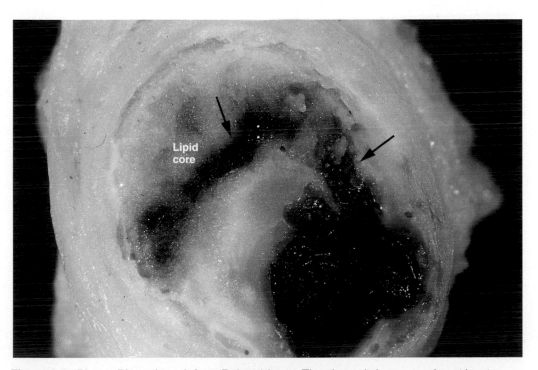

Figure 3-7. Plaque Disruption—Infarct-Related Artery. The plaque is large, causing at least 50% diameter stenosis. In the plaque, a track (*arrows*) leads down into the lipid core but there is not a large intraplaque thrombus. Recent thrombus occludes the arterial lumen.

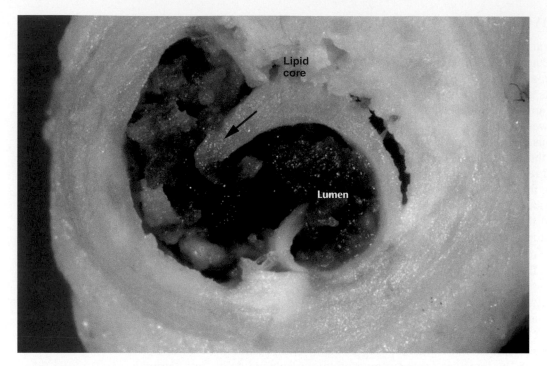

Figure 3-8. Plaque Disruption—Infarct-Related Artery. This plaque with a large lipid core was also causing significant preexisting stenosis. The cap has broken (*arrow*) and there is a mass of thrombus within the plaque in continuity with a mass of thrombus similar in size occluding the lumen.

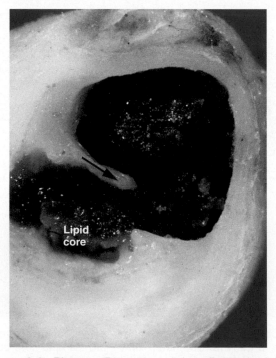

Figure 3-9. Plaque Disruption—Infarct-Related Artery. There was no preexisting stenosis and the end of the torn plaque cap is visible (*arrow*) with thrombus within the lipid core in continuity with thrombus within the arterial lumen.

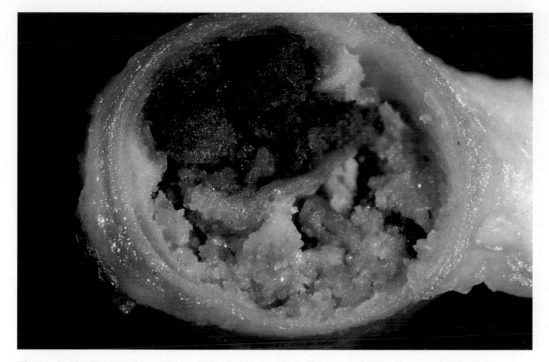

Figure 3-10. Plaque Disruption—Infarct-Related Artery. It is not possible to ascertain if the plaque was causing stenosis because the cap has disintegrated, leaving the artery filled with a mixture of lipid debris released from the core and thrombus.

In a minority of disruption episodes the thrombus is almost entirely within the plaque core itself and the acute obstruction is due to a massive expansion of the plaque from within, without an intraluminal component of thrombus (Fig. 3-11). In endothelial erosion the thrombus is superimposed on the plaque surface and there is no intraplaque component (Fig. 3-12). High-grade stenosis is more consistently related to endothelial erosion thrombi than it is in plaque-disruption–induced thrombi (Fig. 3-13). Some evidence is beginning to emerge that the mechanism by which thrombosis is triggered over a plaque may vary in different patient groups (12). Plaque disruption appears to be the mechanism by which the great majority of males with hypercholesterolemia develop thrombosis. In 59 coronary thrombi causing sudden death in men, 41 were due to disruption and 18 were due to endothelial erosion. The ratio of serum cholesterol to high-density lipoprotein (HDL) cholesterol was 8.5 ± 4.0 in the former, $5.0 \pm$ in the latter. In women (13,14) and diabetic subjects, endothelial erosion may be relatively more important (Table 3-1) than disruption in causing thrombosis. More knowledge is needed on how individual risk factors and gender influence plaque morphology and thus the mechanisms of thrombosis. While plaque disruption has come into prominence in the last decade, it was known to pathologists and clinicians at the end of the last century. George Dock (15) gave an excellent description in 1896. Constantinides (16), however, was largely responsible from 1966 onward for an increasing recognition of the condition that he called plaque fissuring. Once angiography in life had established that the artery supplying the infarct zone was occluded and then reopened and the significance of the type II angiographic lesion was recognized, the role of thrombosis, plaque disruption (rupture), and endothelial erosion was finally fully established.

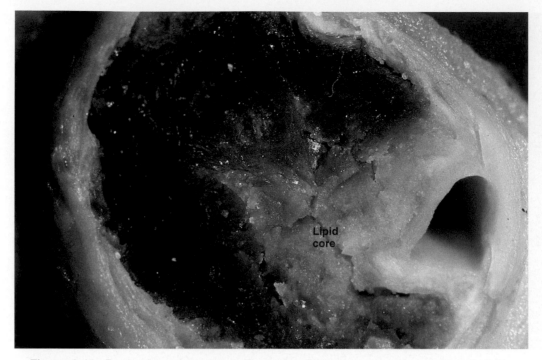

Figure 3-11. Predominant Intraplaque Thrombus. There is a massive expansion of the plaque by a mass of thrombus within the lipid core. A small plaque cap tear was present proximally but in this particular section the cap is intact.

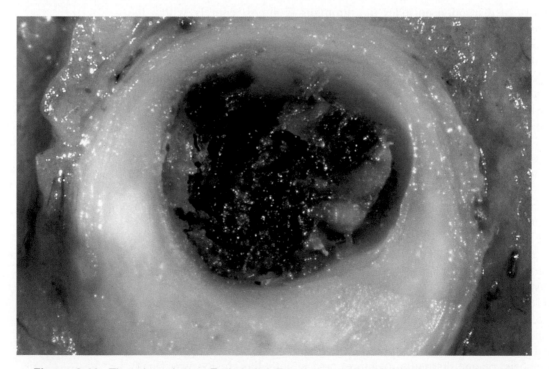

Figure 3-12. Thrombus due to Endothelial Erosion. A mass of thrombus occludes this infarct-related artery. A plaque is present but it shows no thrombus within the core. Preexisting stenosis does not appear to be more than mild.

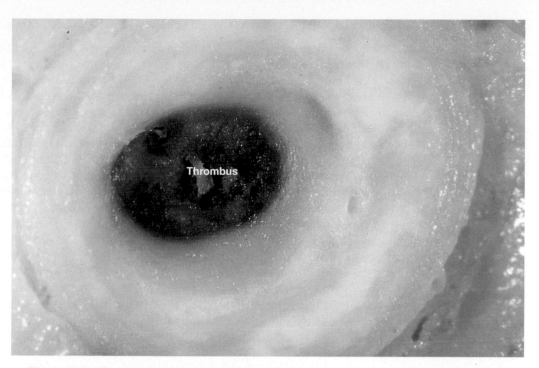

Figure 3-13. Thrombosis due to Endothelial Erosion. There is high-grade stenosis due to a concentric fibrous rather than a lipid-rich plaque. Thrombus occludes the lumen but the plaque is intact.

Table 3-1. *Mechanisms of thrombosis—subgroup variation*

	Plaque disruption	Endothelial erosion
Male (*n*=34)[1]	82%	18%
Male (*n*=134)[2]	84%	16%
Female (*n*=16)[1]	31%	69%
Female (*n*=27)[2]	59%	41%
Diabetic (*n*=41)[2]	34%	66%

[1]From ref. 13
[2]From ref. 14

PLAQUE DISRUPTION AND ACUTE REGIONAL INFARCTION

Disruption (rupture) can only complicate plaques in which there is a lipid core separated from the lumen by a layer of fibromuscular tissue, the plaque cap. When the cap tears, blood enters the core itself where in the first stage of thrombosis a platelet-rich thrombus develops within the plaque, which is expanded and, as a consequence, may rapidly increase the degree of stenosis. Thrombosis may now extend in a second stage to project into but not occlude the lumen, and finally, thrombosis may become occlusive and begin to propagate distally (Fig. 3-14). The second stage of the thrombosis involves both platelets and fibrin, while the third and final occluding stage is rich in fibrin and red cells. The number of platelets in the thrombus within the plaque core itself suggests that blood enters and leaves the core via the cap tear for an appreciable time. In focal areas, large numbers of red cells may also accumulate in the core, giving an appearance sometimes known as plaque hemorrhage. There has been a view that such intraplaque hematomas cause a sudden increase in plaque volume and therefore rapidly increase the degree of stenosis. This undoubtedly occurs (Fig. 3-11), but is not the result of hemorrhage from transmedial vessels entering the base of the plaque. When large intraplaque hematomas are reconstructed in their entirety from serial histological sections, a proximal or distal break in the plaque cap is found. Much of the previous literature concerning the origin of plaque hematomas was based on examining single cross sections of the plaque that did not happen to pass through the tear in the cap.

As emphasized in Figs. 3-7 to 3-11 there is a wide variation in the microanatomy of disrupted plaques that cause major coronary thrombi. At one extreme the cap tear may be minor, the intraplaque component small, yet the thrombus present in the lumen is very large. Such lesions are the type everyone who uses fibrinolytic drugs would like to treat. In the mid-part of the spectrum are lesions in which the intraplaque component and intraluminal components are more matched in size. At the other extreme are lesions in which the major element causing occlusion is expansion of the plaque by thrombus within the core, or where cap tissue and core contents spill out into the arterial lumen. Such complex disruptions are likely to do better with primary angioplasty. The cap tears may be complex with a spiral arrangement lifting intimal flaps or even a proximal entry tear and a distal exit tear. Fibrinolytic therapy is highly efficient in removing the final occluding stage of thrombus, which is highly predictable, given that this element of the occlusion is made up of a loose network of fibrin with enmeshed red cells. The underlying disrupted plaque is, however, then exposed and will be at risk of a further occluding event for some weeks at least (Figs. 3-15, 3-16). The thrombus within the core may become organized into fibrous tissue but the surface is still covered by residual thrombus at 10 days. Thrombus within the core may be lysed and, if the cholesterol has been washed out into the lumen and distributed downstream, a small ulcer crater is left, which can be seen on angiography (Fig. 3-17). Such craters are more common in large arteries, such as the carotid, but do occur in coronary arteries. The culprit lesion both after acute infarction treated by lysis and after unstable angina has a greater risk of thrombosis if the vessel outline remains ragged (complex angiographic lesion) compared with lesions that become smooth in outline (17). Combined therapy with warfarin and aspirin reduces the risk of reocclusion.

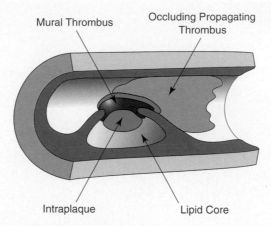

Mural Thrombus   Occluding Propagating Thrombus

Intraplaque   Lipid Core

Figure 3-14. The Different Components of Thrombus after Disruption. The thrombus within the plaque has a large component of platelets, as thrombus begins to project into the lumen the fibrin component becomes more dominant, while the occluding thrombus is made up of a network of fibrin in which there are numerous trapped red cells. Over the surface of the mural thrombus there is also a layer of platelets.

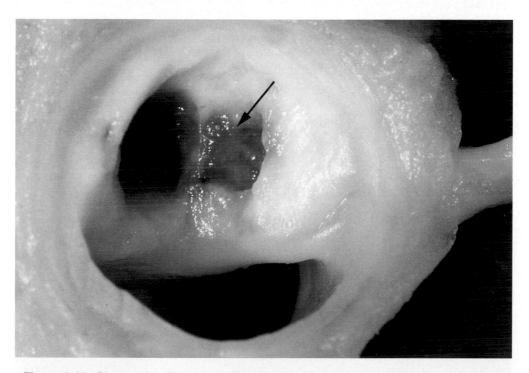

Figure 3-15. Plaque after Fibrinolysis. This plaque was related to an infarct and the patient had been treated with fibrinolytic therapy 10 days before death. The plaque has a crater (*arrow*) in the surface on the floor, of which a layer of residual thrombosis is present. The lumen is patent but narrowed by the upward bulge of the plaque, which is expanded by organizing thrombus within the core.

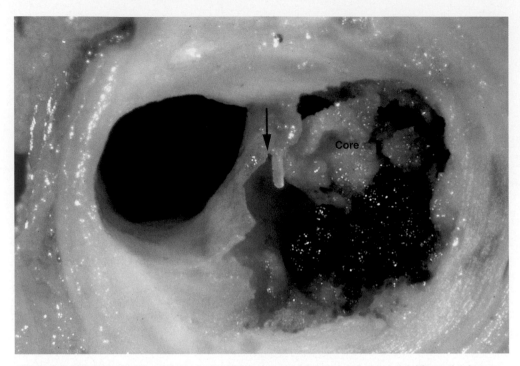

Figure 3-16. Plaque after Fibrinolysis. Thrombus has been totally removed from the lumen of this infarct-related artery but a hole is still present in the plaque cap (*arrow*) and within the core there is residual thrombus. Lysis 5 days before death. It is easy to see why such a lesion has a high risk of recurrent thrombotic occlusion.

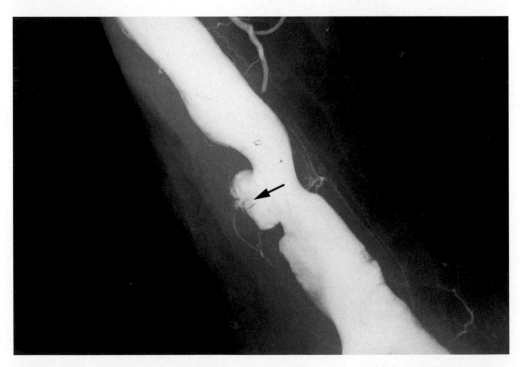

Figure 3-17. Angiographic Crater following Disruption. The angiogram shows a crater (*arrow*) with overhanging edges. This appearance results from plaque disruption after which all the intracore thrombus has been lysed and the cholesterol washed downstream into the intramyocardial vasculature as cholesterol emboli.

ENDOTHELIAL EROSION AND ACUTE REGIONAL INFARCTION

The personal experience of Davies (14), Farb (13), and Burke (12) is that in middle-aged males, endothelial erosion over a plaque is a rare cause of occlusion. The frequency of this form of thrombosis is, however, higher in diabetic subjects, in familial hypercholesterolemia (Fig. 3-18), and perhaps in women. The typical lesion is a concentric intimal thickening packed with foam cells and high-grade stenosis with a final superimposed thrombus.

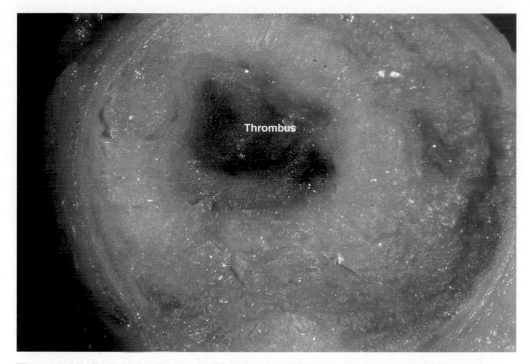

Figure 3-18. Endothelial Erosion in Familial Hypercholesterolemia. In this woman with a total plasma cholesterol of 14.8 ml there is concentric intimal thickening with diffuse deposition of lipid rather than the formation of discrete plaques. The small residual lumen is occluded by thrombus.

UNSTABLE ANGINA

The challenge presented in the understanding of the pathogenesis of unstable angina is the wide spectrum of severity and risk of death or infarction in the patients. The divergence is so great that some clinicians view unstable angina as a mild condition, others as a medical emergency. Broadly defined (18), unstable angina is a clinical syndrome lying between stable angina and acute myocardial infarction. Inherent in the clinical diagnosis are combinations of a recent change in the frequency and nature of pain and/or pain at rest. There is a conceptual problem in that any subject who presents with stable exertional angina must have been symptom-free for 1 week and have symptoms in the next week. All patients with stable angina, therefore, must have had an unstable phase in the past. The term unstable angina is, however, usually reserved for subjects who have at the present time worsening exertional or rest pain and a temporal transitory course, i.e., the patient develops an acute infarct, dies suddenly, or resolves with settling of pain.

A number of classifications have been designed to stratify patients into like groups so that therapeutic trials can be evaluated. Braunwald (19) suggested three groups. In A, sometimes called secondary unstable angina, there is a systemic condition, such as anemia, which intensifies myocardial ischemia. In B, the condition develops suddenly, in the absence of any extra cardiac disease, and in group C, the condition develops after a myocardial infarction. Within each there is a subdivision attempting to adjust for duration and severity. In I there is new onset of angina or a significant change in severity of stable angina, in II there is rest angina within the past month but not in the last 48 hours, and in III there is rest pain for the last 48 hours. The Agency for Health Core Policy and Research (AHCPR) and the National Heart, Lung and Blood Institute (NHLBI) have evolved a rather simpler classification into:

Rest angina—angina at rest within the last week
New onset angina—angina on exertion of at least Canadian Cardiovascular Society
    Classification III severity with onset in the last 2 months
Increasing angina—previous angina that has become more frequent, longer duration,
    and lower threshold in last 2 months with an increase to at least class III severity

The clinical spectrum fits well with the spectrum of pathological changes that occur following plaque disruption (Table 3-1). In effect, unstable angina equates to an unstable plaque that is undergoing thrombosis.

The pathological basis of Braunwald group IIIB resting angina has been the most widely studied, both by clinical methods and at autopsy. Pathological studies were inevitably biased toward the worst possible outcome—death. The advent of atherectomy and angioscopy (20) (Table 3-2), however, has provided valuable additional data in subjects who are still alive.

The initial understanding of the pathogenesis of crescendo resting (Braunwald IIIB) unstable angina came from angiography in life (21). It became apparent that there was a culprit angiographic lesion with very characteristic morphology. These culprit lesions are eccentric, with an irregular outline and may have overhanging edges and intraluminal filling defects suggesting thrombus formation (Fig. 3-19). The angio-

Table 3-2.

Plaque pathology	Clinical symptomology
Predominant intraplaque thrombus	Sudden plaque growth —Silent angiographic progression —Onset or worsening of stable angina on exercise
Intraplaque with nonocclusive mural thrombus projecting into lumen	Unstable angina ↓ Non-Q wave infarction
Intraplaque with occluding lumenal thrombus	Transmural myocardial infarction

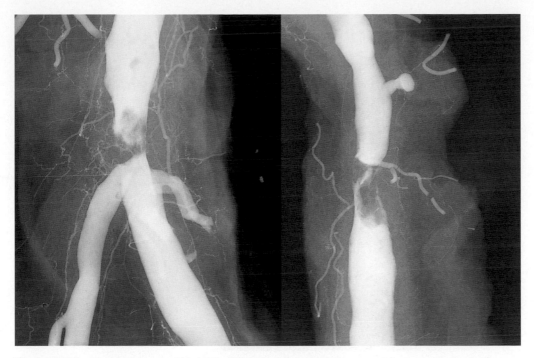

Figure 3-19. Angiography in Unstable Angina. Characteristic eccentric ragged stenoses are present with a small amount of attached intraluminal thrombus.

graphic appearances contrast to the smooth outline of stenoses responsible for stable exertional angina. A seminal pathological angiographic study (6) then showed the basis of the typical culprit lesion was a disrupted plaque with associated thrombus. This was further reinforced by pathological studies of subjects dying suddenly after resting chest pain. The characteristic of the artery in unstable angina is that antegrade flow was still present (Figs. 3-19–3-26). Even postmortem angiograms will not detect more than three quarters of plaques that have thrombosis either due to disruption or erosion. It is, therefore, hardly surprising that angiography *in vivo* does not always identify a culprit lesion in life. It is probably that the unstable nature of the lesions shown in Figs. 3-20 and 3-21 would have been identified *in vivo* by angiography.

As emphasized earlier, the thrombotic response to an episode of plaque disruption is staged. The initial thrombus is within the plaque thrombus then projects into the lumen and finally occludes. Patients with unstable angina are arrested in the second phase and it can be postulated that factors that might cause progression and those that promote the process of lysis and healing are equally balanced.

The typical thrombus of unstable angina (Figs. 3-22–3-26) that projects into but does not occlude the lumen has a base of densely packed fibrin, but the surface is covered by a layer of activated platelets. These platelets have the potential to embolize into the intramyocardial vascular bed (Fig. 3-27). The platelet clumps express the IIb/IIIa receptor very strongly, allowing their identification by immunohistochemistry. Platelet clumps can be identified in intramyocardial arteries over a wide range of sizes. Platelet masses occlude the smaller arteries and are associated with clumps of polymorphonuclear white cells (Figs. 3-28, 3-29). Aggregates of activated platelets can be identified in intramyocardial capillaries and these platelets are likely to pass through into the systemic circulation. Episodic platelet activation can be demonstrated in subjects with unstable angina (22–24). Platelet microthrombi are found only in the segment of myocardium distal to a culprit thrombotic coronary artery lesion. Autopsy studies of subjects dying suddenly after rest pain show at least 50% to have easily demonstrable platelet microemboli, which when present are associated with microscopic foci of

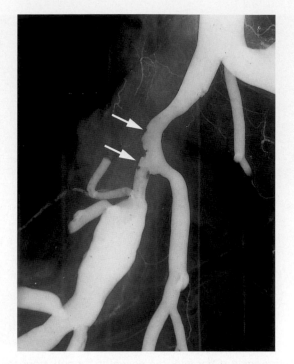

Figure 3-20. Angiogram in Unstable Angina. In contrast to
Fig. 3-19, there is a long segment of artery that is concentri-
cally narrowed with a slightly saw-toothed outline (*arrows*).
These appearances are those of thrombus deposition due to
endothelial erosion in a preexisting stenosis.

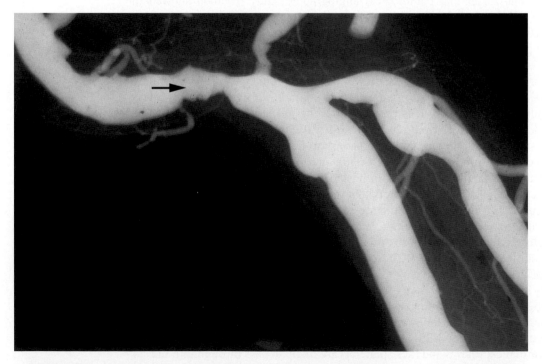

Figure 3-21. Angiogram in Unstable Angina. A segment (*arrow*) can be recognized to have
a slightly irregular outline rather like that in Fig. 3-20, but to a lesser degree. Thrombus was
due to endothelial erosion. It is unlikely this would be recognized as a thrombotic unstable
plaque in an angiogram taken in life.

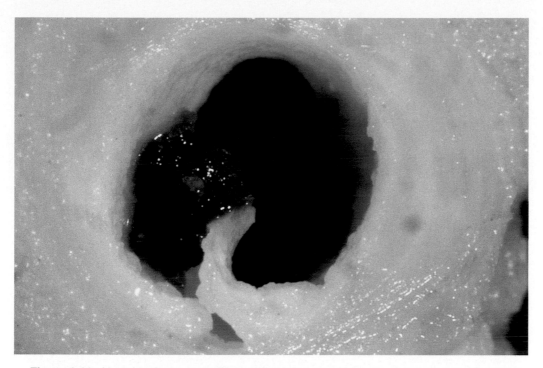

Figure 3-22. Unstable Angina with Plaque Disruption. In this small episode of disruption the plaque cap is torn and projects upward, partially covering a thrombus within the lipid core.

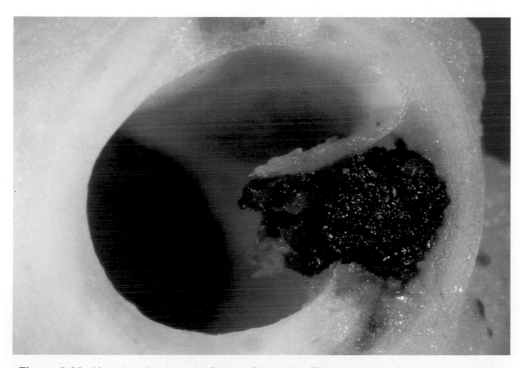

Figure 3-23. Unstable Angina with Plaque Disruption. The plaque cap is torn and projects into the lumen, exposing a mass of thrombus filling the original lipid core of the plaque.

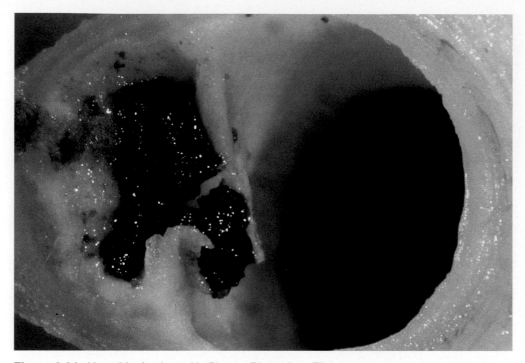

Figure 3-24. Unstable Angina with Plaque Disruption. The appearances are very similar to those in Figs. 3-22 and 3-23, indicating that this is a frequently seen piece of pathology. In Figs. 3-22–3-24 the degree of preexisting stenosis is minimal. Symptoms were presumably due to combinations of spasm, distal emboli, or intermittent growth of the thrombus followed by lysis.

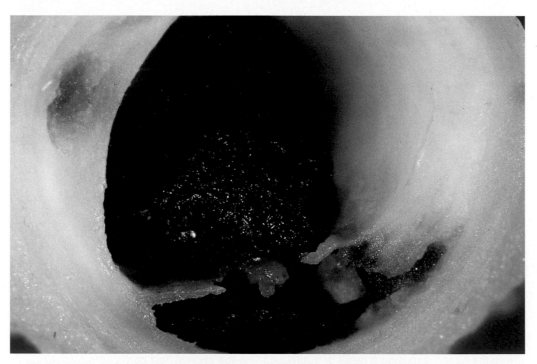

Figure 3-25. Unstable Angina with Plaque Disruption. In this case, the size of both the intraplaque and intraluminal thrombus is far larger than in Figs. 3-22–3-24.

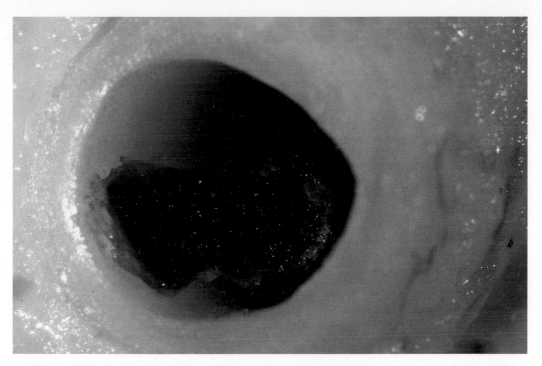

Figure 3-26. Unstable Angina with Plaque Erosion. A pedunculated mass of thrombus with a broad base is adherent to the luminal surface of a plaque that shows no evidence of disruption.

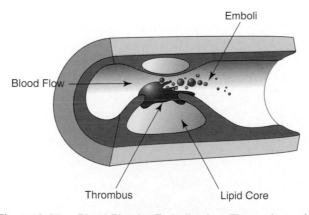

Figure 3-27. Distal Platelet Embolization. The surface of a protruding but nonoccluding thrombus is covered by activated platelets, and aggregates of these may embolize into the distal microvascular bed.

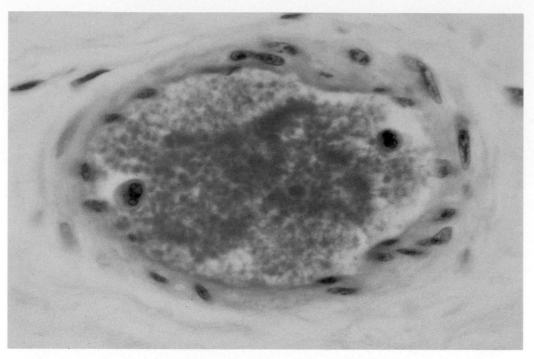

Figure 3-28. Intramyocardial Platelet Emboli. An intramyocardial artery of approximately 700 μm external diameter is blocked by a large mass of aggregated platelets. The section has been treated with an antibody to the platelet 2b/3a receptor. The bright-red staining indicates a high level of expression of the receptor on these platelets.

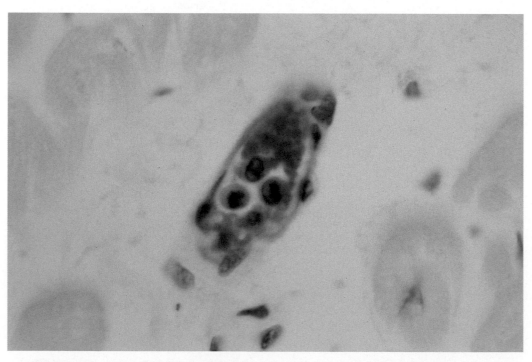

Figure 3-29. Intramyocardial Platelet Emboli. A small intramyocardial artery with an external diameter of 100 μm is blocked by a mass of red-staining platelets and some polymorphs.

myocyte necrosis (Fig. 3-30) (25,26). Local platelet deposition over the culprit plaque may induce spasm, particularly if the lesion is eccentric, leading to intermittent reduction in myocardial blood flow providing a further mechanism for myocardial ischemia (27,28). The relation of sensitive *in vivo* methods, such as Troponin-T levels for showing myocyte necrosis and thus identifying high-risk patients, is therefore explicable (29,30). The clinical perception of unstable angina as a condition without myocardial infarction is a reflection of the low sensitivity of the ECG for the detection of small focal areas of myocyte necrosis.

Atherectomy Studies in Unstable Angina

The advantage of atherectomy studies is that patients with the less severe forms of unstable angina can be studied. The disadvantage is that not all culprit lesions are identified or can be reached and that the sample of the plaque that is removed is a random fragment that may not be representative of the lesion overall. Taken together, the studies published (31–35) have a consistent message:

1. The frequency of thrombus over culprit lesions in unstable angina is higher than lesions associated with stable angina.
2. Some stable plaques associated with stable angina have thrombus in the atherectomy sample.
3. Lipid core material and lipid-filled macrophages are more common in the culprit lesions of unstable angina (36) than those of stable angina.
4. Gelatinase B and Tissue Factor (TF) expression is more common in the plaques causing unstable angina (37,38).

All of these facts are consistent with the hypothesis that unstable angina is caused by unstable plaques with a high lipid and inflammatory cell activity in which thrombosis is occurring. It is clear that these features are not absolute and occur to a lesser

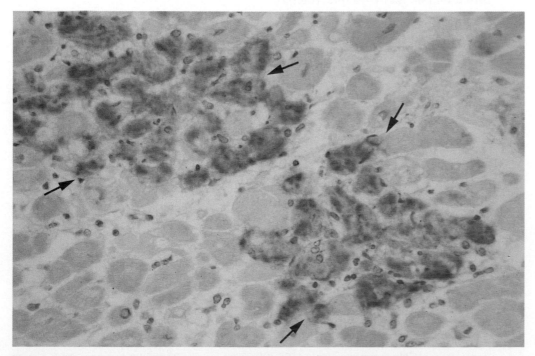

Figure 3-30. Microscopic Infarction in Unstable Angina. The section has been stained by immunohistochemistry to show the binding of the C9 component of complement to two (*red*) foci of myocyte death (*arrows*). The foci of dead myocytes are small and focal fitting into a low-power microscopic field. C9 binding indicates early myocyte necrosis.

degree in many of the plaques responsible for stable angina (39). It is particularly relevant that thrombotic material may be found in apparently clinically stable plaques. Smooth muscle proliferation with a storiform pattern (Fig. 3-33) taken to indicate an accelerated growth phase (40) is seen in unstable angina more frequently than in stable plaques and is discussed in more detail below (see p. 90).

Angioscopy Studies in Unstable Angina

Direct examination of culprit lesions by angioscopy (20) has confirmed much of what was revealed by atherectomy, but the frequency of demonstrating thrombus is higher (Table 3-3), suggesting a greater sensitivity. Culprit plaques are usually yellow, indicating that they have a high lipid content.

Vascular Spasm and Unstable Angina

At the other extreme from the thrombogenic pathogenesis of unstable angina is the concept that pure vascular spasm can occur in localized segments of a coronary artery. Even when these spastic segments are angiographically normal, necropsy and intravascular ultrasound evidence suggests that an atherosclerotic plaque is present (41,42). The reasons why intense excessive vasomotor tonal responses should develop over a particular plaque are unclear. One factor is undoubtedly endothelial dysfunction (43), and there is a possible interaction with microscopic platelet deposition (44). The classic case recorded by Brown et al. (45), in which the abnormal segment of artery was excised, showed such microthrombosis. Alternative suggestions have included release of vasoconstrictor substances from adventitial chronic inflammatory cells (46). There is probably a continual spectrum in unstable angina from cases with pure spasm through cases with thrombosis and spasm to pure thrombosis. Most cases seen in Western countries seem to lie toward the thrombogenic end of the spectrum.

Inflammation and Unstable Angina

In unstable angina in the acute phase of the disease C-reactive protein (CRP) is raised in the plasma (47) and has some predictive value for death or nonfatal infarction. Serum neopterin levels are also raised in unstable angina (48). Neopterin is a macrophage product produced after stimulation by interferon-τ and is elevated in a number of immune-mediated reactions, including allograft rejection. In unstable angina there is also a transient lymphocyte activation (49). There are a number of possible explanations for an acute systemic inflammatory response in unstable angina. Over the culprit coronary artery lesion there will be exposed thrombus covered by a layer of activated platelets. The contact phase of coagulation is activated and remains so for far longer than the acute symptoms (50). Plasma kallikrein levels are elevated, indicating increased bradykinin production, but fall to near normal over 10 days. Fibrinogen levels rise to a maximum on the 5th day and remain elevated. Thrombin antithrombin complexes are elevated. The key factor in such studies is that thrombogenic/fibrinolytic activity continues long after the clinical condition of the patient has settled.

Table 3-3. *Angioscopy in angina*

	Unstable	Stable
Thrombus	70 (73.7%)	4 (14.8%)
No thrombus	25 (26.3%)	23 (85.2%)
	95 (100%)	27 (100%)

From ref. 20.

As emphasized previously, unstable angina is associated with embolization of clumps of activated platelets into the distal myocardial bed and plugging of small vessels by polymorphs occurs. Microscopic foci of myocyte necrosis are far more common than clinically appreciated. Such foci will in themselves invoke acute inflammation. Elevation of plasma Troponin-T levels is seen in up to 35% of patients with unstable angina, and such patients have an increased risk of further cardiac reflecting of this microvascular damage (29,30,51). The risk is incremental as plasma Troponin-T levels are elevated.

It is, therefore, not a surprise that there is evidence of a systemic inflammatory reaction in the acute phase of unstable angina. The most interesting observations are, however, that markers of inflammatory activation may precede and predict unstable angina. In the European Concerted Action on Thrombosis (ECAT) trial (52), the levels of CRP, while not elevated above normal, predicted acute events over 3 years. CRP levels, however, correlate with other risk factors, such as age, smoking, cholesterol, triglycerides, and body mass index as well as with serological evidence of chlamydia and helicobacter infection (53). One explanation of these facts is that CRP reflects the general level of inflammatory activity in plaques within an individual and the higher this activity is the more likely that vulnerable plaques are present and, therefore, the greater the risk of an acute event. The Physicians' Trial of Aspirin showed that the upper quartile of individuals with the highest CRP gained the greatest benefit from aspirin (Table 3-4) (54). This could be explained by the fact that this quartile had the majority of acute thrombotic events and would, therefore, most benefit.

Table 3-4. *Physicians' Health Study of Aspirin—Risk of myocardial infarction*

Quartiles of plasma—C-reactive protein	Risk
1 Low	1.16
2	2.07
3	2.59
4 High	4.16

From ref. 54.

ATHEROSCLEROTIC DISEASE PROGRESSION

Clinical studies define progression both in terms of the number of new acute ischemic episodes that occur and in terms of the progression of lesions in successive angiograms. Angiographic analysis often separates new chronic totally occlusive lesions not associated with recognized episodes of infarction, increase in the degree of stenosis in preexisting high- or medium-grade lesions and the appearance of "new" lesions in segments of artery that were normal at the previous examination. The term *new* must not be confused with the initiation of a new plaque. The plaque that has appeared has probably been there for at least some years but has finally reached the threshold where it begins to encroach on the lumen and become visible. Studies of the natural history of coronary disease show that angiographic progression and the new acute ischemic event counts correlate with each other, i.e., they represent to a large degree a common process (55,56). The most likely mechanism are cycles of thrombosis and repair within plaques. The lessons learned from sequential angiograms (57–60) are:

1. Progression is intermittent and step-like.
2. High-grade stenotic lesions do develop from the slow progression of preexisting lesions, but it is also very common for high-grade lesions to appear *de novo* between two angiograms.
3. Many chronic total occlusions occur in previously normal arterial segments.
4. It is impossible from the angiogram to predict where thrombotic episodes will occur—many develop over minor stenoses or in normal segments of artery.

Silent Plaque Disruption

A number of pathological studies (Table 3-5) have suggested that episodes of plaque disruption are relatively common events and are often clinically silent (7,61,62). In subjects who have died of an acute ischemic event, it is usually possible to identify a major culprit lesion, though there are often other smaller acute plaque events in the same patients (Fig. 3-31). In subjects with coronary disease but who die of other noncardiac causes, small plaque disruption can be found (Fig. 3-32) (63).

Healing of Plaque Disruption

The healing response to an episode of plaque disruption is an attempt to both restore the vascular lumen and to restabilize the plaque (also see Chapter 4). Thrombotic material is removed by either natural or therapeutic fibrinolytic activity. This process seems most effective for thrombotic material in the original lumen, less so for thrombus within the original lipid core of the plaque. Thrombotic material that is not removed invokes a florid smooth muscle proliferation in which there is a storiform pattern of cells arranged in a loosely arranged matrix (Fig. 3-33). Collagen synthesis begins and ultimately restores a smooth outline and restores plaque stability. The reparative process has varying degrees of success and may produce anything from a chronic fibrotic total occlusion (see Chapter 4) to virtually no increase in the degree of stenosis from that previously present (Figs. 3-34–3-36). If thrombus has persisted

Table 3-5. *Coronary disease progression—silent disruption is common*

Davies (63)
    110 subjects with noncardiac sudden death, 16 (14.5%) had a small recent plaque disruption
Falk (86), Frink (62)
    130 subjects with coronary disease and sudden death
    314 disruption episodes—2.4 per subject

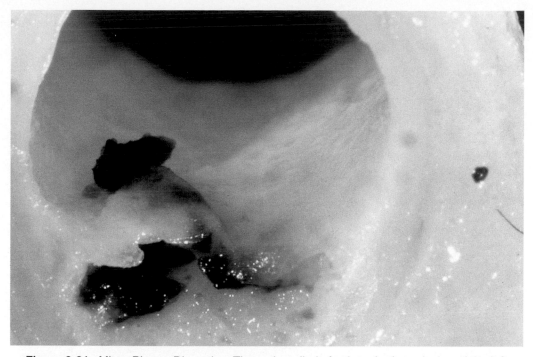

Figure 3-31. Minor Plaque Disruption. The patient died of a thrombotic occlusion of the left anterior descending coronary artery. In the right coronary artery there was this additional small recent plaque rupture.

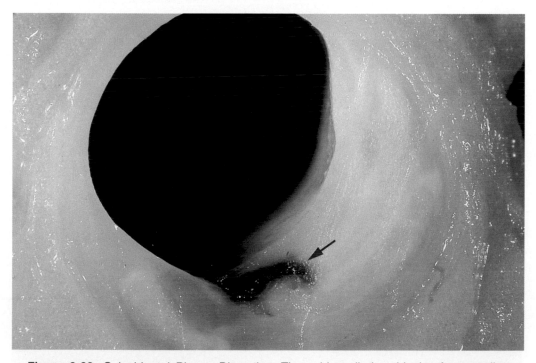

Figure 3-32. Coincidental Plaque Disruption. The subject died suddenly of noncardiac causes. At the edge of a lipid-rich plaque there is a fissure with an entirely intraplaque small hematoma (*arrow*).

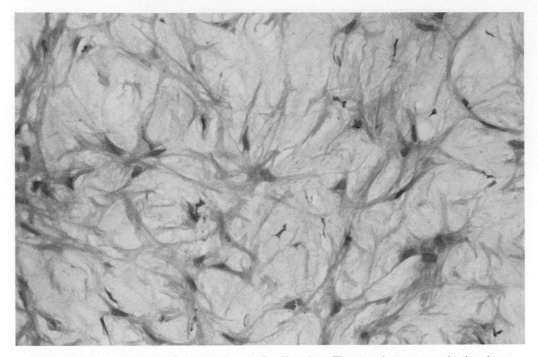

Figure 3-33. Accelerated Smooth Muscle Proliferation. The repair response in the damaged plaque is of smooth muscle proliferation in which the cells are arranged in a characteristic storiform pattern. The smooth muscle cells are separated by the abundant connective tissue matrix they produce. In the early stages this is largely proteoglycans, which are then replaced by collagen (hematoxylin and eosin).

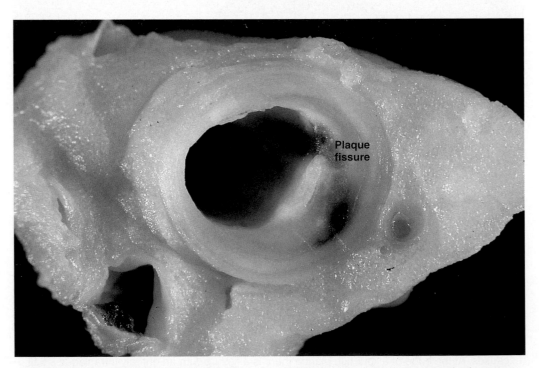

Figure 3-34. Healed Recent Plaque Disruption. There is still some recent thrombotic material in the plaque tissue but there is development of gray material (*arrow*), which is newly formed connective tissue that is beginning to replace the thrombus and fill in the core. The degree of stenosis has not been appreciably increased.

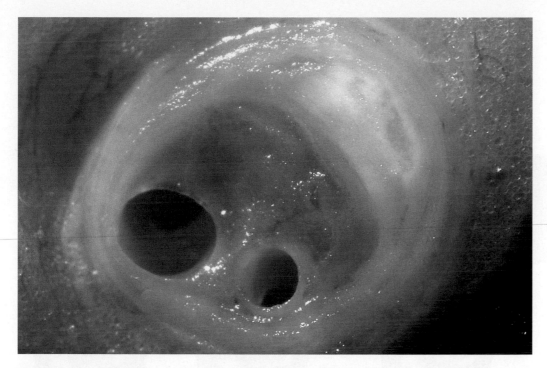

Figure 3-35. Healed Plaque Disruption. The lumen is largely filled with gray, recently formed connective tissue within which there are two new vascular lumens. Resolution of the process here has been ineffective in restoring a large lumen.

in the lumen it may be replaced by smaller vessels (Fig. 3-35). The speed of the process of repair is unclear, but probably takes some weeks or months. Clinical data suggests that with a disrupted plaque in which flow is restored by lysis in patients with impending infarct there is a high risk of further occlusion for some weeks, which then slowly declines over months. Where the lipid content of the core has been washed out after loss of the whole cap a small crater is left that appears like an aneurysm in the angiogram (Fig. 3-17). The long-term future of these craters is unknown in the coronary arteries. Such craters are far more common in larger arteries such as the aorta and carotids and do become reendothelialized with time.

Atherectomy studies in unstable angina that show an accelerated smooth muscle proliferation pattern (40) are most logically explicable by the sample being taken from a disrupted plaque that has entered its repair phase. Our own studies (35) show a consistent relation of this histological pattern to Braunwald IIB unstable angina.

The Vulnerable Plaque Concept and Lipid-Lowering Therapy

The advent of effective lipid-lowering drugs of the statin group, which were well tolerated by patients and have a good safety profile, has led to four major trials—the Scandinavian Simvastatin Survival Study (4S) (64), CARE (65), WOSCOPS (66), and the LIPID study, which have a consistent message. The pooled data in four pravastatin trials designed originally to show angiographic regression showed a similar reduction in acute events (67). Lipid lowering significantly reduces the risk of future acute ischemic events and thereby reduces all cause mortality. Previous angiographic trials of lipid lowering had shown that there was an affect on chronic stenosis but this was minimal; new angiographic lesion appearance was, however, reduced (68). A logical explanation of these facts is that lipid lowering in some way alters plaque biology to reduce the risk of thrombosis.

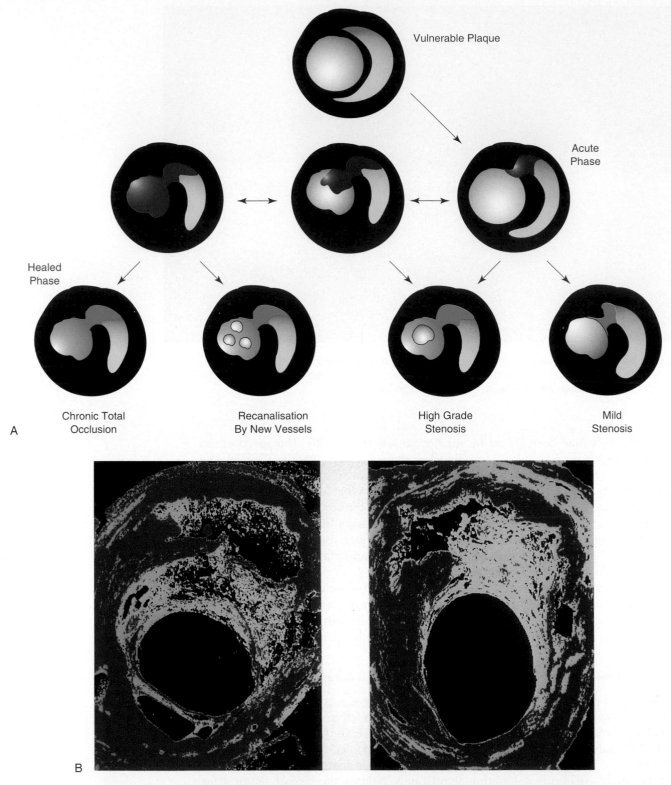

Figure 3-36. The Potential Outcome of Plaque Disruption. **A.** The outcome of an episode of plaque thrombus depends on how rapidly thrombus is lysed and how rapidly and to what extent new collagen deposition occurs. (*Thrombus, red; connective tissue, green.*) **B.** The cross sections of two arteries have been color-coded to show newer collagen in yellow, older collagen in red. One artery **(left)** was related to a prior infarct and shows considerable encroachment on the lumen by new fibrous tissue and a fibrous strand crossing the lumen. The non-scar–related artery **(right)** shows new connective tissue filling in the disrupted plaque and extending around part of the lumen to some degree.

Pathology studies of atherosclerosis suggest that patients with coronary atherosclerosis have a varying number of plaques. The number of plaques (total plaque burden) will be a measure of the risk of a future event. Patients also vary widely (69) in the proportion of their plaques, which are at high risk of undergoing disruption or erosion, i.e., they are vulnerable (Table 3-6). The major components of the plaque-conferring vulnerability are a large lipid core, a thin cap, and a high inflammatory activity based on the number of activated macrophages. Many plaques in the stable state have some of these characteristics and, as stressed by Becker (39), plaque vulnerability is a variable relative factor. High risk occurs when all the factors coincide (70). The future risk of an acute event in any individual subject with ischemic heart disease is directly related to the number of vulnerable plaques, not the total number of plaques overall. The ratio between vulnerable and nonvulnerable plaques, which could be called a "vulnerability index," is, however not presently determinable *in vivo*. The increasing evidence that systemic markers of inflammatory activity are indicators of prognosis, however, may be indicating that it is possible to determine those subjects with many inflammatory plaques. The differing numbers of vulnerable plaques between individuals is the explanation for why some subjects have one infarct and remain symptom-free for years while other less fortunate individuals have a new ischemic event annually. An important corollary of the vulnerable plaque concept is that while angiography is an excellent indicator of the present state of the coronary arteries, it does not and cannot indicate the risk of future events. There is no correlation of the features conferring vulnerability with angiographic stenosis (71).

The mechanisms by which lipid lowering reduces vulnerability have to a large extent been studied in experimental models of atherosclerosis using the Watanabe rabbit and high-lipid diets in both rabbits and primates. There is a consistent picture of a decline in the number of foam cells and activated macrophages and an increase in the number of smooth muscle cells within plaques, culminating in the plaque becoming more solid and fibrous (72–74).

Table 3-6. *The vulnerable plaque concept—*
variation in plaque characters in subjects who had stable angina

Percent of all plaques with a lipid core	Number of Individuals	
0–10% (Low vulnerability)	9	16.7%
11–40%	16	29.6%
41–70%	17	31.5%
71–100% (High vulnerability)	12	22.2%
Total	54	100%

From ref. 69.

ACUTE ISCHEMIC SYNDROMES: THE MYOCARDIAL LESIONS

Clinicians and pathologists often have different perspectives on the usage of the term *myocardial infarction*. The term strictly means any myocardial necrosis that is due to reduction or interference with the oxygen availability to the myocyte. Within such a definition there are a number of forms of myocardial infarction having very different pathophysiological mechanisms (Fig. 3-37). To the clinician the term myocardial infarction usually implies a regional area of myocardial necrosis that can be recognized and localized by the ECG. This implies a disease, usually thrombosis due to atherosclerosis, in the epicardial artery supplying that segment of myocardium. Other far rarer causes of regional infarction include spasm, spontaneous dissection, myocardial bridging, emboli, etc. The pathologist can recognize histologically, areas of necrosis as small as a few myocytes, especially if immunohistochemical techniques are used (Fig. 3-31). These foci are too small to produce ECG changes. Clinicians and pathologists differ in their sensitivity for detecting infarction and hence do not always agree on the answer to the question—"Did this patient have a myocardial infarction?"

Human Regional Infarction

The dog models of myocardial infarction in which sudden ligation of a coronary artery produces a regional area of myocardial necrosis provided a wealth of data on the mechanisms and pathophysiology of infarction (75,76), which have influenced think-

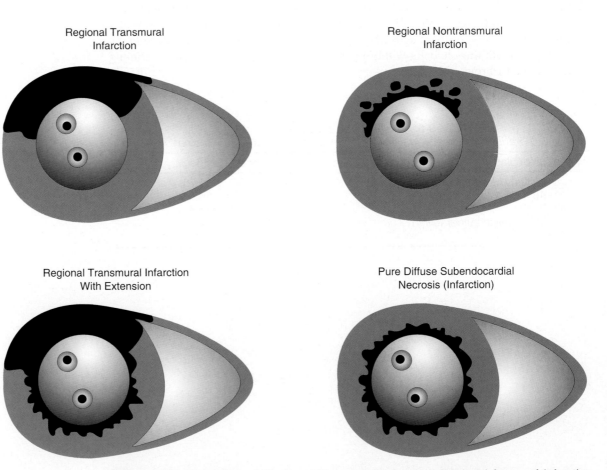

Regional Transmural
Infarction

Regional Nontransmural
Infarction

Regional Transmural Infarction
With Extension

Pure Diffuse Subendocardial
Necrosis (Infarction)

Figure 3-37. The Different Forms of Myocardial Infarction. Regional forms of infarction reflect a pathological or pathophysiological mechanism in the coronary artery supplying that particular segment of the ventricular myocardium. Diffuse, nonregional infarction is usually due to a fall in overall myocardial perfusion and is maximal in the subendocardial zone.

ing concerning human lesions to a major degree. The simplicity of the model does however tend to obscure the fact that human thrombotic occlusions cover a far wider range of time relations. At one extreme, the plaque disruption is sudden and major, leading to thrombotic occlusion within a short time. At the other extreme, the thrombosis is stuttering in onset, with intermittent occlusions and reflow over some days before final occlusion. In unstable angina there is a risk of total occlusion developing, but before this stage, platelet emboli into the myocardium occur. The result of the variable onset of thrombotic occlusion in human disease is that there is a wide spectrum of morphology in human regional infarcts.

In regional transmural infarction the usual finding is that of necrosis of a uniform age (Fig. 3-38). The subtending artery at autopsy is usually occluded totally with distal extension of thrombus. The far higher frequency of such totally occluded arteries in pathology studies when compared with clinical angiographic studies suggests a selection bias indicating the poor prognostic factor of persistent occlusion.

Pathologists use histochemistry to demonstrate the loss of enzymes from infarcted myocardium, but this technique is useful in defining the pattern of necrosis (Fig. 3-39) rather than its early detection. In contrast to transmural infarction, regional nontransmural infarction is rarely of a uniform age histologically and in enzyme-stained preparations appears built up from smaller foci of myocyte necrosis of widely differing age (Fig. 3-40). This form of infarction is now more common at autopsy than the uniform transmural type. At least part of the evolution of nontransmural infarction is due to microscopic foci of necrosis associated with distal platelet emboli, another potential cause is intermittent occlusion in the epicardial artery in question. Nontransmural infarction is the characteristic lesion of those subjects who progress to non-Q wave infarction from unstable angina. The clinical terms *Q* and *non-Q wave infarction* are broadly but not exactly synonymous with the pathological terms *transmural* and *nontransmural*. Discrepancies arise because of the insensitivity of the ECG for small areas

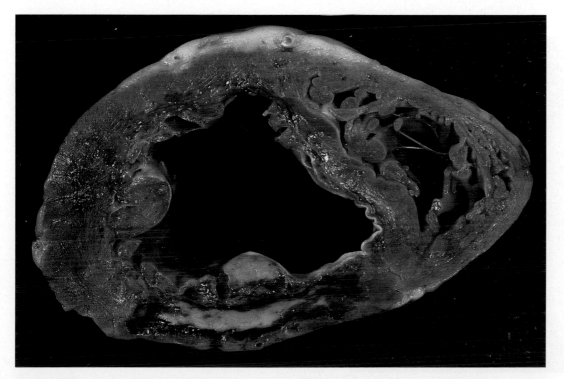

Figure 3-38. Human Regional Infarction. In this traditional pathologist's view of infarction in a patient dying 6 days after the onset of chest pain there is a transmural, sharply defined zone of yellow necrotic muscle with a red rim on the posterior wall of the left ventricle.

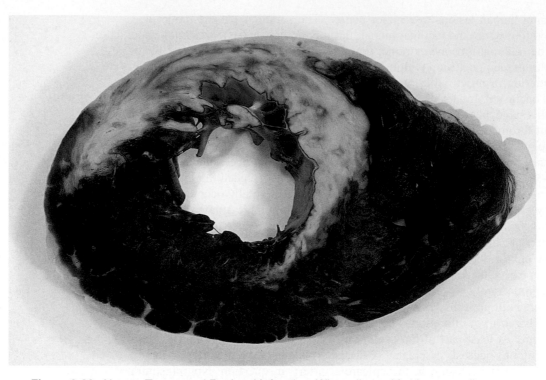

Figure 3-39. Human Transmural Regional Infarction. When slices of fresh myocardium are incubated with succinate and the dye Nitro BT, areas in which there is succinate dehydrogenase enzyme appear dark blue. Areas of infarction in which the dehydrogenase enzymes are lost appear unstained. This myocardial slice shows a transmural anteroseptal infarct. In the septal area the infarct has a nontransmural component, while in the anterior wall it is transmural. The very discrete sharp lateral borders of infarcts following ligation of a coronary artery in the dog are rare in humans.

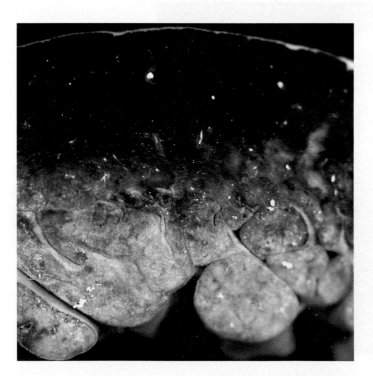

Figure 3-40. Human Nontransmural Infarction. The subepicardial zone is viable and maintains its deep blue color reaction showing normal enzyme activity. The subendocardial zone shows total enzyme lost. In the mid-zone there are focal areas of partial enzyme loss intermingled with focal normal areas.

of transmural extension in a predominantly nontransmural infarct. The essential differences between Q and non-Q wave infarction is the high frequency of complete occlusion in the former, while in the latter antegrade blood flow in the supplying artery is maintained (77,78) either by rapid lysis of thrombus, by collateral flow, or by the thrombus remaining nonocclusive due to the exact balance of forces leading to its growth or its resolution. Unstable angina of Braunwald type IIIB represents a patient suspended in limbo for some days with exposed thrombus in a coronary artery that is neither growing or resolving. If the balance tips toward more thrombosis, the characteristic infarct is nontransmural.

It is not the role of this book to discuss in detail the complex microscopic changes that pathologists use to attempt to identify infarction at microscopy. There are, however, a few salient points for clinicians to be aware of.

Pathologists cannot identify with certainty myocardial infarction by histological methods unless the patient has survived the onset of infarction by at least 12 to 18 hours. More sophisticated methods, such as the identification of the membrane attack complex of complement (C9) on myocytes by immunohistochemistry, can reduce the time interval for recognition but are not widely used. The usual mode of necrosis seen in infarcts of uniform age involves a sequence of morphological changes. The myocyte swells as fluid enters the dying cell, the myofibrils begin to disintegrate and the nucleus vanishes. The cell breaks up and is removed by macrophages after which fibrosis begins. These changes occur most rapidly at the border of the infarct with viable myocardium. If flow is restored to an already established regional infarction, intense interstitial bleeding occurs leading to a hemorrhagic macroscopic appearance.

In infarcts in which there are foci of necrosis of rather different age representing combinations of embolic damage and intermittent restoration of flow, a different form of necrosis occurs. In this contraction-band necrosis (Fig. 3-41) there is intense hyper-

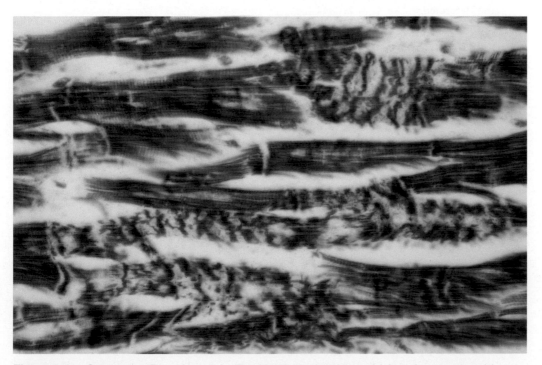

Figure 3-41. Contraction Band Necrosis. The histological stain used (phosphotungstic acid hematoxylin) shows myofibrils as dark blue. In the upper portion of the picture are myocytes showing the normal appearance with regular cross striations. In the lower portion of the picture the myofibrils have condensed into irregular masses.

contraction of the myofibrils within the myocyte, giving a characteristic cross-banding appearance (79–81). The changes result from restoring blood flow to myocytes in which ischemic damage has increased permeability to calcium ions. The sudden influx of calcium causes intense myofibrillary contraction. Because the changes occur very rapidly it is a sensitive and early method of pathological detection of myocardial infarction, but occurs only in situations where reperfusion has occurred. These histological changes are also very common in infarcts reperfused by thrombolysis; in these cases there is also intense interstitial hemorrhage.

Nonregional Human Infarction

Pathologists recognize diffuse nonregional subendocardial myocardial necrosis as resulting from a wide variety of causes, all of which have a common pathophysiological mechanism in a fall of overall myocardial perfusion. Necrosis involves the subendocardial zone and the centers of the papillary muscles. The process begins as foci of necrosis and may coalesce and culminate in complete necrosis of the whole inner third of the circumference of the left ventricle. Diffuse subendocardial necrosis will complicate regional infarction when cardiogenic shock occurs and is one form of infarct extension. Patients with cardiogenic shock (82) enter a spiral of poor myocardial perfusion leading to subendocardial necrosis leading to a further fall in myocardial perfusion. Diffuse subendocardial necrosis is seen in many conditions where the epicardial coronary arteries are morphologically normal and is accentuated by both pressure and volume overload hypertrophy. End-stage severe aortic valve stenosis, for example, is associated with subendocardial necrosis even in the absence of coronary disease. Modern out-of-hospital resuscitation is producing more examples of this form of myocardial necrosis following long resuscitation intervals before cardiac output is restored. The majority of patients who are on a respirator for some days after resuscitation will have both raised intercranial pressure and diffuse subendocardial myocardial necrosis.

COMPLICATIONS OF MYOCARDIAL INFARCTION

Serious structural complications of infarcts are almost entirely found after transmural infarction. External cardiac rupture is responsible for approximately 10% of infarct mortality. Two distinct forms of rupture exist (83). In one there is a slit or tear through the ventricular wall at a stage before the actual infarct is easily visible at autopsy. The infarct is not expanded (Fig. 3-42) and the tear occurs at the margin of the viable tissue, probably due to shear stresses set up at the interface between beating and nonbeating muscle. This form of rupture characteristically occurs in the first 36 hours after the onset of pain. At this stage, infiltration by polymorphs is present in the border of the infarct. The second and rarer form of rupture occurs later, after onset, and is essentially a complication of infarct expansion (Figs. 3-43–3-45). The rupture is usually a jagged-edged hole at the apex of a distinct bulge in the ventricle. There is usually local pericarditis. Infarct expansion is a complication of transmural infarcts in which the necrotic myocardium thins and bulges outward. This process does not involve new necrosis, just a change in shape of the infarct zone due to tearing and slippage of myocytes relative to each other. Expansion is strikingly related to large transmural infarcts and is usually found following persistent occlusion of the left anterior descending coronary artery above the first septal perforator. Ventricular septal defects may also complicate acute infarcts that have or have not expanded. Papillary muscle infarction is very common, complicating at least 40% of posteroinferior infarcts and rather less of anterior infarcts. Papillary muscle infarction heals by fibrosis, leading ultimately to mild mitral regurgitations. Papillary muscle rupture due to infarction (Fig. 3-46) is rare (84), found in less than 1% of fatal myocardial infarcts. Papillary muscle rupture is not necessarily confined to transmural or large infarcts. A distinct entity exists of a nontransmural infarction of the anterolateral papillary muscle due to thrombosis in the left marginal artery.

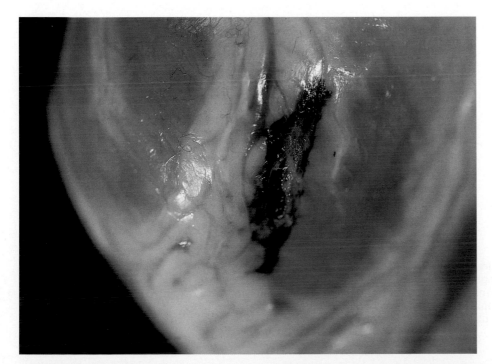

Figure 3-42. Early External Cardiac Rupture. Viewed from the epicardial surface the rupture is a slit-like tear not associated with infarct expansion or acute pericarditis.

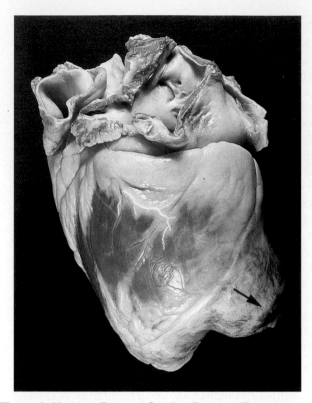

Figure 3-43. Late External Cardiac Rupture. There is a very marked external bulge as seen from the epicardial surface. Rupture occurred at the apex of the bulge (*arrow*).

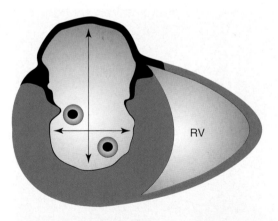

Infarct Expansion

Figure 3-44. Infarct Expansion. Infarct expansion is a change in shape of an existing infarct and does not involve new necrosis. The infarct thins and the ventricular cavity becomes asymmetric, with very different distances in short axis planes taken at right angles.

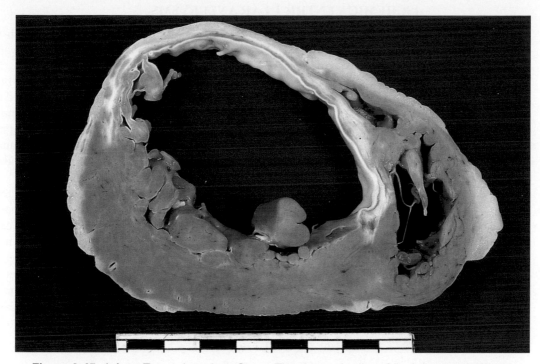

Figure 3-45. Infarct Expansion—Late Stage. The short axis slice of the left ventricle shows a healed expanded anteroseptal infarct in which there is a fixed outward bulge. The surviving myocardial tissue on the posterior and lateral wall of the ventricle has undergone hypertrophy.

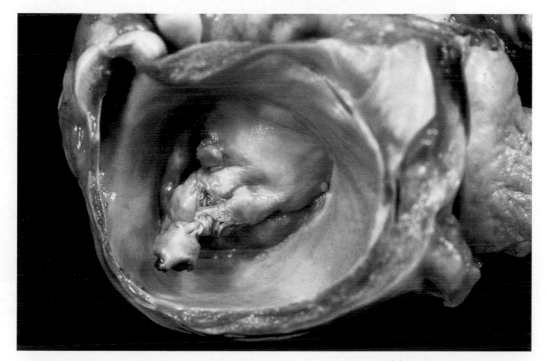

Figure 3-46. Ischemic Papillary Muscle Rupture. Viewed from the left atrium at necropsy the stump of the papillary muscle can be seen to have been prolapsing across the mitral valve.

ISCHEMIC VENTRICULAR ANEURYSMS

Traditionally, distinction is made between true aneurysms, in which the wall is derived from the myocardium itself, and false aneurysms, in which the wall of the sac is derived from pericardium. True aneurysms have a wide neck (Fig. 3-47), false aneurysms have a narrow neck that opens into a large external sac (85) (Fig. 3-48). True aneurysms derive from fibrosis of an acute infarct that has expanded and usually develop within 10 days of the onset of pain. In the fully evolved infarct, thrombus may or may not be present on the endocardium. The rim of the fully evolved infarct develops white endocardial thickening and buried in this fibrous tissue are anastomosing strands of surviving subendocardial myocytes. These myocardial strands provide a structural basis for reentry tachycardias.

The origin of what are called pseudoaneurysms is rather different. They represent the end stage of a partial rupture of the left ventricle in which a hematoma is confined by the pericardium. The wall of the aneurysm sac is thus made up of pericardial tissue alone. Pathological studies, however, show that this simple dichotomy into true and pseudoaneurysms is not really valid. There is a complete spectrum between aneurysms with a wide neck to those with a narrow aperture opening into a large external sac. The wall nearly always contains both residual myocardium and pericardium. The risk of late rupture in aneurysms with a large external sac and narrow aperture is said to be higher than diffuse aneurysms but the numbers reported are small and inevitably highly selected.

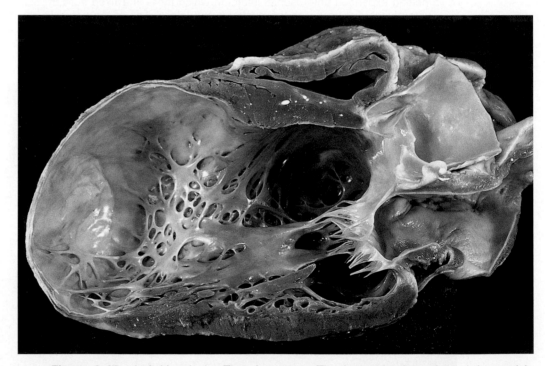

Figure 3-47. Left Ventricular True Aneurysm. The long-axis view of the left ventricle shows a large apical aneurysm with a wide neck. Such aneurysms represent the final stage of infarct expansion.

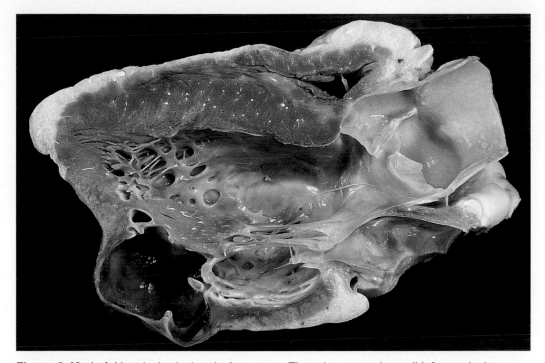

Figure 3-48. Left Ventricular Ischemic Aneurysm. There is a posterior wall left ventricular aneurysm that opens into the left cavity by a relatively small aperture.

REFERENCES

1. DeWood M, Spores J, Notske R, et al. Prevalence of total coronary occlusion during the early hours of transmural myocardial infarction. *N Engl J Med* 1980;303:897–902.
2. Stadius M, Maynard C, Fritz J. Coronary anatomy and left ventricular function in the first 12 hours of acute myocardial infarction: The Western Washington randomized intracoronary streptokinase trial. *Circulation* 1985;72:292–301.
3. Davies M, Woolf N, Robertson W. Pathology of acute myocardial infarction with particular reference to occlusive coronary thrombi. *Br Heart J* 1976;38:659–664.
4. Kim C, Braunwald E. Potential benefits of late reperfusion of infarcted myocardium. The open artery hypothesis. *Circulation* 1993;88:2426–2436.
5. Ambrose J, Winters S, Arora R. Angiographic evolution of coronary artery morphology in unstable angina. *J Am Coll Cardiol* 1986;7:474–478.
6. Levin D, Fallon J. Significance of the angiographic morphology of localized coronary stenosis: histopathologic correlations. *Circulation* 1982;66:316–320.
7. Davies MJ, Thomas A. Thrombosis and acute coronary artery lesions in sudden cardiac ischaemic death. *N Engl J Med* 1984;310:1137–1140.
8. Davies M, Thomas A. Plaque fissuring the cause of acute myocardial infarction, sudden ischaemic death and crescendo angina. *Br Heart J* 1985;53:363–373.
9. Chapman I. The cause effect relationship between recent coronary artery occlusion and acute myocardial infarction. *Am Heart J* 1974;87:267–271.
10. Fulton FM. Pathological concepts in acute coronary thrombosis: relevance to treatment. *Br Heart J* 1993;70:459–470.
11. Henriksson P, Edhag O, Jansson B. A role for platelets in the process of infarct extension. *N Engl J Med* 1985;313:1660–1661.
12. Burke A, Farb A, Malcom G, Liang Y-H, Smialek J, Virmani R. Coronary risk factors and plaque morphology in men with coronary disease who died suddenly. *N Engl J Med* 1997;336:1276–1282.
13. Farb A, Burke AP, Tang AK, et al. Coronary plaque erosion without rupture into a lipid core, a frequent cause of coronary thrombosis in sudden coronary death. *Circulation* 1996;93:1354– 1363.
14. Davies MJ. The composition of coronary-artery plaques. *N Engl J Med* 1997;336:1312–1314.
15. Dock G. Notes on the coronary arteries. In: Mauer AK, Mauer EF, eds. *George Dock, MD: A bibliography of his writings*. Los Angeles: Barlow Society for the History of Medicine of the library of the Los Angeles County Medical Association, 1991.
16. Constantinides P. Plaque fissures in human coronary thrombosis. *J Atheroscler Res* 1966;6:1–17.
17. Chen L, Chester M, Redwood S, Huang J, Leatham K, Kaski J. Angiographic stenosis progression and coronary events in patients with "stabilised" unstable angina. *Circulation* 1995;91:2319–2324.
18. Crawford M. Overview. In: Crawford M, ed. *Unstable angina diagnosis and management*. London: Chapman and Hall, 1996:1–24.
19. Braunwald E. Unstable angina, a classification. *Circulation* 1989;80:410–414.
20. White CJ, Ramee SR, Collins TJ, et al. Coronary thrombi increase PTCA risk. Angioscopy as a clinical tool. *Circulation* 1996;93:253–258.
21. Ambrose J, Winters S, Stern A, et al. Angiographic morphology and the pathogenesis of unstable angina. *J Am Coll Cardiol* 1985;5:609–616.
22. Fitzgerald D, Roy L, Catella F, Fitzgerald A. Platelet activation in unstable coronary disease. *N Engl J Med* 1986;315:983–989.
23. Fitzgerald D, Roy L, Catella F, FitzGerald G. Platelet activation in unstable angina. *J Am Coll Cardiol* 1987;10:998–1004.
24. Hamm C, Lorenz R, Bleifeld W, Kupper W, Wober W, Weber P. Biochemical evidence of platelet activation in patients with persistent unstable angina. *J Am Coll Cardiol* 1987;10:998–1006.
25. Falk E. Unstable angina with fatal outcome: dynamic coronary thrombosis leading to infarction and/or sudden death. *Circulation* 1985;71:699–708.
26. Davies M, Thomas A, Knapman P, Hangartner R. Intramyocardial platelet aggregation in patients with unstable angina suffering sudden ischaemic cardiac death. *Circulation* 1986;73:418–427.
27. Yao S, Ober J, Benedict C, et al. ADP plays an important role in mediating platelet aggregation and cyclic flow variations *in vivo* in stenosed and endothelium-injured canine coronary arteries. *Circ Res* 1992;70:39–48.
28. Hamm CW, Ravkilde J, Gerhardt W, et al. The prognostic value of serum troponin T in unstable angina. *N Engl J Med* 1992;327:146–150.
29. Stubbs P, Collinson P, Moseley D, Greenwood T, Noble M. Prospective study of the role of cardiac troponin T in patients admitted with unstable angina. *BMJ* 1996;313:262–264.
30. Lindahl B, Venge P, Wallentin L, FRISC Study G. Relation between Troponin T and the risk of subsequent cardiac events in unstable coronary artery disease. *Circulation* 1996;93:1651–1657.
31. Rosenschein U, Ellis SG, Haudenschild CC, et al. Comparison of histopathologic coronary lesions obtained from directional atherectomy in stable angina versus acute coronary syndromes. *Am J Cardiol* 1994;73:508–510.
32. Escaned J, van Suylen RJ, MacLeod DC, et al. Histologic characteristics of tissue excised during directional coronary atherectomy in stable and unstable angina pectoris. *Am J Cardiol* 1993;71:1442–1447.
33. Hofling B, Welsch U, Heimer J, et al. Analysis of atherectomy specimens. *Am J Cardiol* 1993;72:96E–107E.
34. Waller BF, Johnson DE, Schnitt SJ, et al. Histologic analysis of directional coronary atherectomy samples. *Am J Cardiol* 1993;72:80E–87E.
35. Mann JM, Kaski JC, Arie S, et al. Plaque constituents in patients with stable and unstable angina: an atherectomy study. *J Am Coll Cardiol* 1995;27:240A(abst).
36. Moreno P, Falk E, Palacios, et al. Macrophage infiltration in acute coronary syndromes: implications for plaque rupture. *Circulation* 1994;90:775–778.

37. Annex B, Dennings S, Channon K, et al. Differential expression of tissue factor protein in directional atherectomy specimens from patients with stable and unstable coronary syndromes. *Circulation* 1995;91:619–622.
38. Brown D, Hibbs M, Kearney M, et al. Identification of 92-kD gelatinase in human coronary atherosclerotic lesions: association of active enzyme synthesis with unstable angina. *Circulation* 1995;91:2125–2131.
39. van der Wal AC, Becker AE, Koch KT, et al. Clinically stable angina pectoris is not necessarily associated with histologically stable atherosclerotic plaques. *Heart* 1996;76:312–316.
40. Flugelman MY, Virmani R, Correa R, et al. Smooth muscle cell abundance and fibroblast growth factors in coronary lesions of patients with nonfatal unstable angina. A clue to the mechanism of transformation from the stable to the unstable clinical tool. *Circulation* 1993;88:2493–2500.
41. Roberts WC, Curry RC, Isner JM. Sudden death in Prinzmetal's angina with coronary spasm documented by arteriography: analysis of three necropsy cases. *Am J Cardiol* 1982;50:203–210.
42. Yamagishi M, Miyatake K, Tamai J. Intravascular ultrasound detection of atherosclerosis at the site of focal vasospasm in angiographically normal or minimally narrowed coronary segments. *J Am Coll Cardiol* 1994; 23:352–357.
43. Zeiher AM, Goebel H, Schachinger V, et al. Tissue endothelin-1 immunoreactivity in the active coronary atherosclerosis plaque: A clue to the mechanism of increased vasoreactivity of the culprit lesion in unstable angina. *Circulation* 1995;91:941–947.
44. Lam JY, Chesebro JH, Steele PM, et al. Is vasospasm related to platelet deposition: relationship in a porcine preparation of arterial injury *in vivo*. *Circulation* 1987;76:243–248.
45. Brown B, Bolson EL, Dodge HT. Dynamic mechanisms in human coronary stenosis. *Circulation* 1984;70: 917–922.
46. Kohchi K, Takebayashi S, Hiroki T, Nobuyoshi M. Significance of adventitial inflammation of the coronary artery in patients with unstable angina: results at autopsy. *Circulation* 1985;71:709–716.
47. Liuzzo G, Biasucci L, Gallimore J, et al. The prognostic value of C-reactive protein and serum amyloid. A protein in severe unstable angina. *N Engl J Med* 1994;331:417–424.
48. Gupta S, Fredericks S, Schwartzman R, Holt D, Kaski J. Serum neopterin is elevated in acute coronary syndromes. *Lancet* 1997;349:1252–1253.
49. Sernery G, Abbate R, Gori A, et al. Transient intermittent lymphocyte activation is responsible for the instability of angina. *Circulation* 1992;86:790–797.
50. Hoffmeister H, Jur M, Wendel P, Heller W, Seipel L. Alterations of coagulation and fibrinolytic and Kallikrein-Kinin systems in the acute and postacute phase in patients with unstable angina pectoris. *Circulation* 1995;91:2520– 2527.
51. Antman E, Tanasikevic M, Thompson B, et al. Cardiac-specific troponin I levels to predict the risk of mortality in patients with acute coronary syndromes. *N Engl J Med* 1996;335:1342–1349.
52. Thompson SG, Kienast J, Pyke SD, et al. Hemostatic factors and the risk of myocardial infarction or sudden death in patients with angina pectoris. European Concerted Action on Thrombosis and Disabilities Angina Pectoris Study Group. *N Engl J Med* 1995;332:635–641.
53. Mendall MA, Goggin PM, Molineaux N, et al. Relation of *helicobacter pylori* infection and coronary heart disease. *Br Heart J* 1994;71:437–439.
54. Ridker PM, Cushman M, Stampfer MJ, et al. Inflammation aspirin and the risk of cardiovascular disease in apparently healthy men. *N Engl J Med* 1997;336:973–979.
55. Waters D, Craven T, Lesperance J. Prognostic significance of progression of coronary atherosclerosis. *Circulation* 1993;87:1067–1075.
56. Azen S, Mack W, Cashin-Hemphill L, et al. Progression of coronary artery disease predicts clinical coronary events. Long-term follow-up from the cholesterol lowering atherosclerosis study. *Circulation* 1996;93:34–41.
57. Bruschke A, Kramer J, Bal E, Haque I, Detranto R, Goormastic M. The dynamics of progression of coronary atherosclerosis studied in 168 medically treated patients who underwent coronary arteriography three times. *Am Heart J* 1989;117:296–305.
58. Lichtlen P, Nikutta P, Jost S, et al. Anatomical progression of coronary artery disease in humans as seen by prospective, repeated, quantitated coronary angiography. Relation to clinical events and risk factors. *Circulation* 1992;86:828–838.
59. Ambrose J, Tannenbaum M, Alexopoulos D, et al. Angiographic progression of coronary artery disease and the development of myocardial infarction. *J Am Coll Cardiol* 1988;12:56–62.
60. Haft J, Haik B, Goldstein J, Brodyn N. Development of significant coronary artery lesions in areas of minimal disease. A common mechanism for coronary disease progression. *Chest* 1988;94:731–736.
61. Falk E. Plaque rupture with severe pre-existing stenosis precipitating coronary thrombosis. Characteristics of coronary atherosclerotic plaque underlying fatal occlusive thrombi. *Br Heart J* 1983;50:127–131.
62. Frink R. Chronic ulcerated plaques: new insights into the pathogenesis of acute coronary disease. *J Invasive Cardiol* 1994;6:173–185.
63. Davies M, Bland J, Hangartner J, Angelini A, Thomas A. Factors influencing the presence or absence of acute coronary artery thrombi in sudden ischaemic death. *Eur Heart J* 1989;10:203–208.
64. 4S Group. Randomised trial of cholesterol lowering in 4444 patients with coronary heart disease: The Scandinavian Simvastatin Survival Study (4S). *Lancet* 1994;344:1383–1389.
65. Sacks F, Pfeffer M, Moye L, et al. The effect of pravastatin on coronary events after myocardial infarction in patients with average cholesterol levels. *N Engl J Med* 1996;335:1001– 1009.
66. Shepherd J, Cobbe S, Ford I, et al. Prevention of coronary heart disease with pravastatin in men with hypercholesterolemia. *N Engl J Med* 1995;333:1301–1307.
67. Byington R, Jukema W, Salonen J, et al. Reduction in cardiovascular events during pravastatin therapy. *Circulation* 1995;92:2419–2425.
68. Jukema J, Bruschke A, van Boven A, et al. Effects of lipid lowering by pravastatin on progression and regression of coronary artery disease in symptomatic men with normal to moderately elevated cholesterol levels: the Regression Growth Evaluation Statin Study (REGRESS). *Circulation* 1995;91:2528–2540.
69. Hangartner J, Charleston A, Davies M, Thomas A. Morphological charactertistics of clinically significant coronary artery stenosis in stable angina. *Br Heart J* 1986;56:501–508.

70. Davies M. Stability and instability: two faces of coronary atherosclerosis: the Paul Dudley White lecture 1995. *Circulation* 1996;94:2013–2020.

71. Mann J, Davies M. Vulnerable plaque: relation of characteristics to degree of stenosis in human coronary arteries. *Circulation* 1996;94:928–931.

72. Small D, Bond M, Waugh D, Prack M, Sawyer J. Physicochemical and histological changes in the arterial wall of non-human primates during progression and regression of atherosclerosis. *J Clin Invest* 1984;73: 1590–1605.

73. Kaplan J, Manuck S, Adams M, Williams J, Register T, Clarkson T. Plaque changes and arterial enlargement in atheroscleroti monkeys after manipulation of diet and social environment. *Arterioscler Thromb Vasc Biol* 1993;13:254–263.

74. Shiomi M, Tsukaka T, Yata T, et al. Reduction of serum cholesterol levels alters lesional composition of atherosclerotic plaques. Effect of pravastatin sodium on atherosclerosis in mature WHHL rabbits. *Arterioscler Thromb Vasc Biol* 1995;15:1938–1995.

75. Jennings R, Steenbergen CJ, Reimer K. Myocardial ischemia and reperfusion. In: Schoen F, Gimbrone MJ, ed. *Cardiovascular pathology clinicopathologic correlations and pathogenetic mechanisms.* Baltimore: Williams & Wilkins, 1995:47–80.

76. Reimer K, Jennings R, Cobb F. Animal models for protecting myocardium—results of the NHLBI co-operative study. *Circ Res* 1985;56:651–665.

77. DeWood M, Spores J, Notske R. Non-transmural (subendocardial) myocardial infarction in man; the prevalence of total coronary occlusion. *Am J Cardiol* 1981;47:459.

78. Piek J, Becker A. Collateral blood supply to the myocardium at risk in human myocardial infarction: A quantitative post-mortem assessment. *J Am Coll Cardiol* 1988;11:1290–1296.

79. Karch SB. Billingham ME. Myocardial contraction bands revisited. *Hum Pathol* 1986;17:9–13.

80. Hopster D, Milroy C, Burns J, Roberts N. Necropsy study of the association between sudden cardiac death, cardiac isoenzymes and contraction band necrosis. *J Clin Pathol* 1996;49:403–406.

81. Virmani R, Farb A, Burke A. Contraction-band necrosis: new use for an old friend. *Lancet* 1996;347: 1710–1711.

82. Alonso D, Scheidr S, Post M, Killip T. Pathophysiology of cardiogenic shock, quantifications of myocardial necrosis, clinical pathologic and electrocardiographic correlations. *Circulation* 1973;48:588–596.

83. Becker A, van Mantgem J. Cardiac tamponade: a study of 50 hearts. *Eur J Cardiol* 1975;3:349–358.

84. Barbour D, Roberts W. Rupture of a left ventricular papillary muscle during acute myocardial infarction. Analysis of 22 necropsy patients. *J Am Coll Cardiol* 1986;8:548–565.

85. van Tassel R, Edwards J. Rupture of the heart complicating myocardial infarction. Analysis of 40 cases including nine examples of left ventricular false aneurysm. *Chest* 1972;61:104–106.

86. Falk E, Shah PK, Fuster V. Coronary plaque disruption. *Circulation* 1995;92:657–671.

4

Stable Angina

INTRODUCTION

Stable exertional angina is the result of chronic stenotic lesions (Fig. 4-1) in the major epicardial coronary arteries that become flow-limiting on excercise when vascular resistance falls in the distal vascular bed. The practical experience of the many years in which the angiogram has been the major investigative tool of coronary artery disease shows that 50% diameter stenosis is the level at which symptoms may develop. This is also in accord with the hemodynamics that apply to the flow of fluids, with a viscosity similar to that of blood, in tubes *in vitro*.

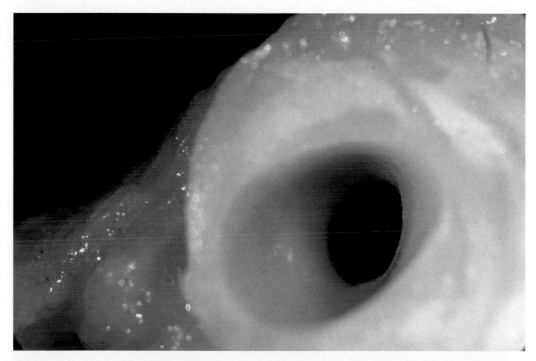

Figure 4-1. Chronic Coronary Stenosis. The coronary artery orifice has a smooth white constriction that narrows the lumen by approximately 60%, as compared with the proximal segment of the artery.

MEASUREMENT OF CORONARY STENOSIS

The measurement of diameter stenosis from angiograms imposes sufficient challenges to raise the question of whether absolute lumen measurements or some assessment of blood flow should be adopted (1). Any measurement of an angiogram necessitates a comparison of the dimensions of the target stenotic segment with an adjacent reference segment, which is judged to be normal on the basis of having a smooth outline (Fig. 4-2). Such reference segments may or may not be normal and, if unrecognized atherosclerosis is present, could either be reduced or increased in diameter. Intravascular ultrasound has firmly established that angiographically normal segments of artery do harbor occult plaques (2–4). The measurement of stenosis makes the assumption that the lumen is close to circular in outline, although *in vivo*, two angiographic views at right angles to each other are usually taken to exclude marked asymmetry of the shape of the lumen. In pathological samples that have been fixed by perfusing the artery at systemic pressures, the lumen does lie very close to being circular in shape. This is confirmed by *in vivo* intravascular ultrasound images. The crescentic and slit-like lumens that are so prominently illustrated in pathology texts are artifacts of collapsed nondistended arteries. There are two major exceptions to this general rule. One exception is where thrombus projects into the lumen when a crescentic-shaped orifice can be produced (Fig. 4-3). The second exception is in plaques that are situated eccentrically, thus leaving a segment of normal vessel wall. The normal segment has a curved outline, while the surface of the plaque itself is often flat, giving a D-shape to the lumen (Fig. 4-4). Whether this shape occurs *in vivo*, and whether the lumen shape changes with the degree of arterial tone is not known. Despite all these potential limitations, simple assessment of angiograms has stood the test of time. The introduction of computer programs to outline the vessel using edge-detection algorithms

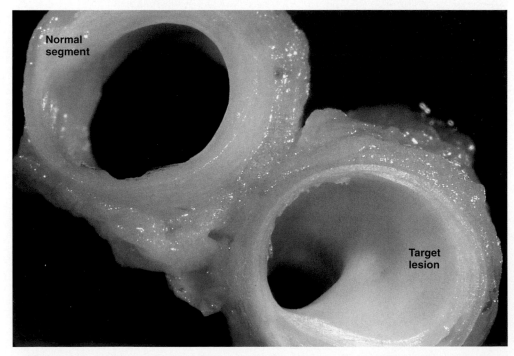

Figure 4-2.   Chronic Coronary Stenosis. The target lesion is a smooth, white narrowing of the coronary lumen; in measuring stenosis the lumen area or diameter at the narrowest point is compared with the lumen of the adjacent normal segment of artery.

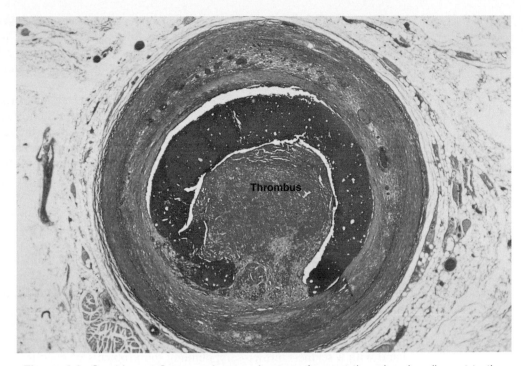

Figure 4-3. Semi-Lunar Coronary Lumen. A mass of recent thrombus is adherent to the arterial wall and protrudes into the lumen. The result is that the residual lumen is crescentic in shape. The lumen contains angiographic medium that appears dark gray in tissue sections.

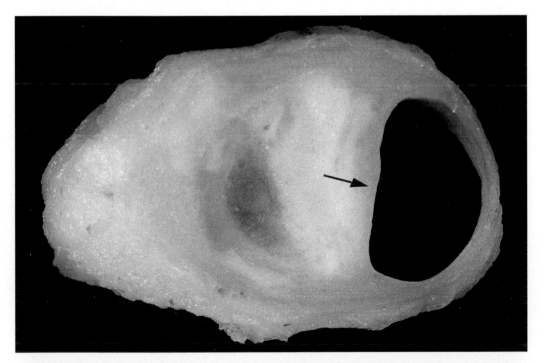

Figure 4-4. D-Shaped Coronary Lumen. Plaques that contain a high proportion of collagen even when the artery is perfused at systemic pressure do not appear to be pliable enough to adopt a lunar shape curved outward and the surface of the plaque has a straighter edge (*arrow*) than the curvature of the normal arterial segment opposite the plaque.

removes any subjective observer bias when very precise measurements of lumen size are needed. Change over time is probably best followed by using absolute dimensions of the test segment to avoid any error due to change in the reference segment. All comparisons *in vivo* at different times make the assumption that vasomotor tone is at the same level.

Pathologists have their own set of challenges when measuring coronary stenosis. The usual method they adopt is to visually assess the degree of stenosis at the test segment using the external diameter of the artery at the same site as the reference value. The comparisons can be made visually or by quantificative measurement of histological slides. The pathology methods totally ignore the phenomenon of compensatory dilatation (remodeling) of the artery in atherosclerosis (see Chapter 2) in which the external diameter in the abnormal segment is often, but not invariably increased. The result is that pathologists consistently and variably overcall stenosis by up to 50% of diameter, as compared with angiographic methods (5). Many papers have stressed that severe limitations of pathologic examination of the coronary arteries leads to erroneous overestimation or underestimation of the degree of luminal narrowing that existed in life (6–8). The best measurement by pathologists would be to compare the target lumen dimensions to an adjacent segment of artery without disease in perfused fixed arteries. The vast majority of necropsy reports, however, rely on subjective naked-eye assessment of cross sections of the unfilled coronary artery in which the lumen has collapsed. Calcification often distorts the cross sections, which are cut freehand with a scalpel, further compounding the problems of quantification. Considerable amounts of time are often spent in legal cases or clinocopathological conferences trying to reconcile the different degrees of stenosis recorded by an angiogram in life and by a necropsy report. The time is largely wasted in trying to reconcile the irreconcilable.

MORPHOLOGY OF STENOSIS IN STABLE ANGINA

Many stenotic segments viewed from the lumen in pathology specimens are smooth white constrictions (Figs. 4-1, 4-2)—this has been confirmed by angioscopy in life. In both ante- and postmortem angiograms, smooth constrictions with a regular outline are frequent, these contrast to the more irregular outlines of the lesions responsible for unstable angina (9). Postmortem angiography, because it has no limits on the exposure time or dose of x-rays, coupled with a lack of movement in the arteries, allows high-contrast, high-definition pictures to be made. While the detail far exceeds that obtainable *in vivo*, certain basic facts about stenosis morphology can be learned. Stenosis in the angiogram can be eccentric or concentric and relatively localized, or extend over a considerable length of the artery (Figs. 4-5–4-9). The feature common to all stable plaques, i.e., not associated with thrombosis, is their smooth outline in the angiogram.

Relatively simple stenoses do have, however, considerable variation in histological structure. Any plaque may be eccentric, i.e., leaving a segment of normal arterial wall opposite the plaque, or be concentric (Figs. 4-10–4-13) without any residual normal arterial wall. Even when there is concentric intimal disease, the residual arterial lumen is, however, not necessarily in the center of the original arterial lumen. Eccentricity in the angiogram does not, therefore, necessarily indicate the presence of a segment of arterial wall capable of vascular tonal responses. Variation in lumen size due to vascular tone changes is, however, a feature of a proportion of stenoses that are eccentric in the angiogram (10,11). The retention of an arc of normal vessel wall is more common in plaques that are not causing significant stenosis (12).

Short segments of stenosis may be caused by single plaques that have nothing to suggest they have arisen by anything more than primary atherogenesis, i.e., lipid accumulation and smooth muscle proliferation. In such plaques, there is a very wide variation in the relative proportion of collagen and lipid within the plaque (Figs. 4-14–4-18) (13). Some plaques have lipid cores, others do not. In any individual, the

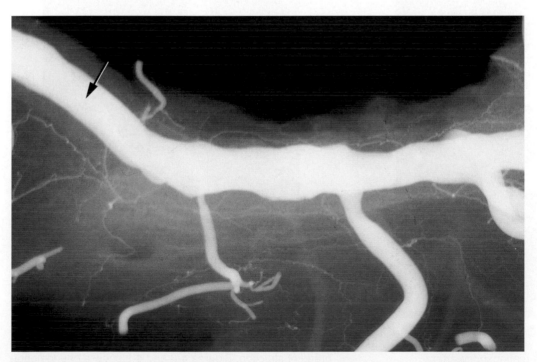

Figure 4-5. Angiographic Coronary Atherosclerosis. In this artery there is no significant stenosis. The presence of numerous plaques is shown by the irregular outline of the lumen in the mid and right-hand segments of the artery. There is a smooth-edged normal segment in the proximal portion of the artery (*arrow*).

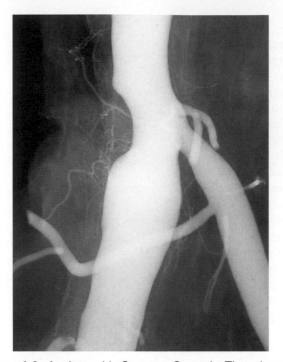

Figure 4-6. Angiographic Coronary Stenosis. There is a discrete eccentric single stenosis (20%) by diameter. The segment of artery distal to the stenosis is larger in diameter (mild ectasia) than the proximal segment illustrating the difficulty in deciding the reference point when calculating angiographic stenosis.

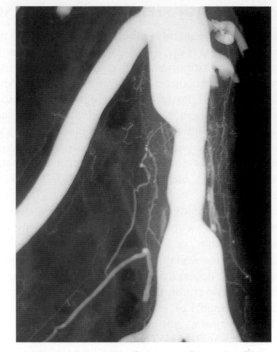

Figure 4-7. Angiographic Coronary Stenosis. There is a 55% diameter concentric stenosis over a 1-cm-long segment of the artery.

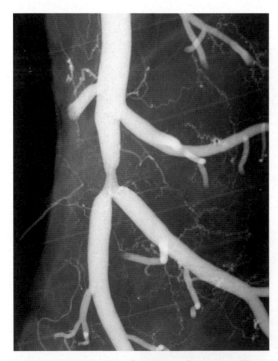

Figure 4-8. Angiographic Coronary Stenosis. There is a high-grade (70% diameter) stenosis due to concentric narrowing just proximal to a bifurcation in the artery.

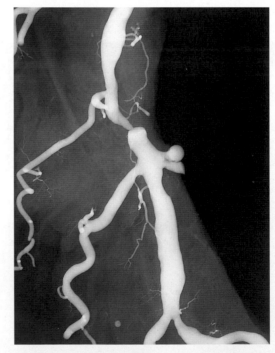

Figure 4-9. Angiographic Coronary Stenosis. There is a very discrete shelf-like concentric stenosis causing very high-grade obstruction. Figures 4-8 and 4-9 show a phenomenon that is also seen in angiography in life—at the stenosis the angiographic media is reduced in density. The pathologist, however, has the distinct advantage that histology can exclude this as being due to thrombus within the lumen.

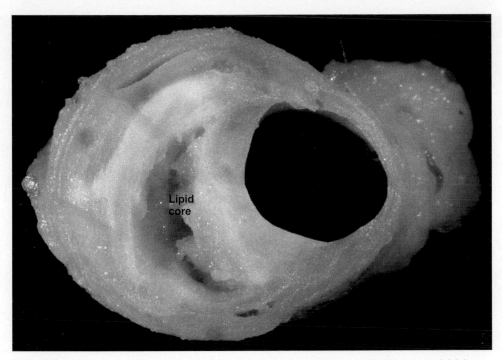

Figure 4-10. Eccentric Coronary Stenosis. This plaque with a large lipid core and thick cap is situated eccentrically, occupying only half of the circumference of the artery. An arc of 180% of normal vessel wall is present opposite the plaque. The degree of stenosis was mild (30% diameter), although the plaque is large, indicating that here was a considerable degree of compensatory dilation on the part of this arterial segment.

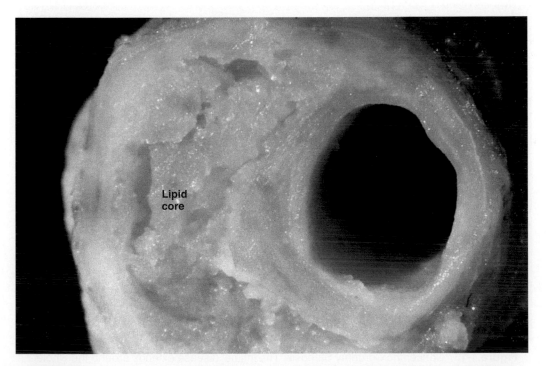

Figure 4-11. Eccentric Coronary Stenosis. The degree of stenosis (52%) was higher than that in Fig. 4-10. The plaque has a large lipid core and a thick cap. The arc of normal artery wall occupies an arc of approximately 150 degrees.

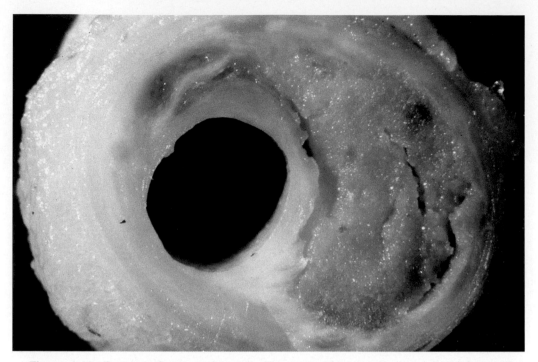

Figure 4-12. Eccentric Coronary Stenosis. There is a high degree of stenosis (70%) and although the main bulk of the plaque is eccentric and the lumen is not placed centrally to the main axis of the artery, intimal disease extends around the whole circumference of the artery and there is no arc of normal vessel wall.

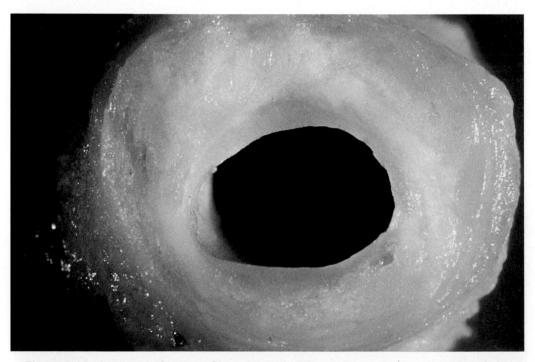

Figure 4-13. Concentric Coronary Stenosis. The intimal disease extends around the whole circumference of the artery, leaving no normal vessel wall. The lumen is central to the long axis of the artery.

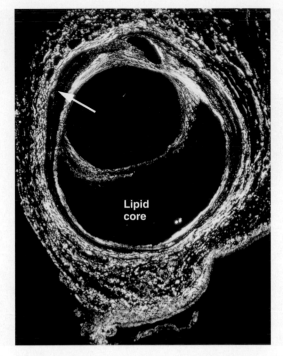

Figure 4-14. Collagen and Lipid in Plaques. The dye Sirius Red binds specifically to collagen and has the property of giving a range of yellow, red, and green colors, depending on the degree of cross linking when viewed under polarized light. The image generated is very similar to intravascular ultrasound images. The media (*arrows*) is a translucent zone due to its being predominantly smooth muscle. The collagen of the plaque and adventitia shows up brightly. In this plaque the lumen is round and the plaque semilunar in shape. The center of the plaque occupied by the lipid core contains no collagen and is a translucent zone. The cap of this plaque is relatively thin.

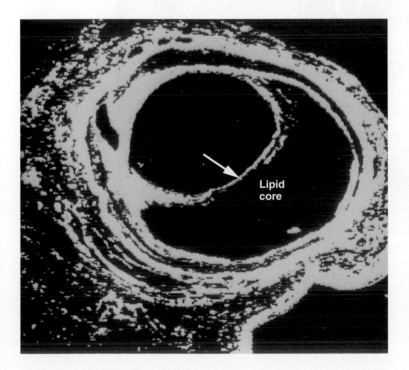

Figure 4-15. Collagen and Lipid in Plaques. The image created by Sirius Red is ideal for scanning into automated quantifying image analysis systems and the image shows all collagen in yellow. The image of the plaque collagen highlights the collagen-free lipid core and the thin plaque cap (*arrow*).

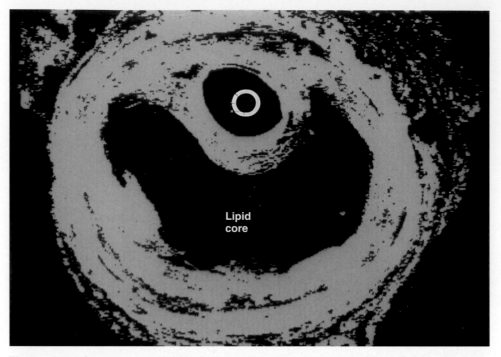

Figure 4-16. Collagen and Lipid in Plaques. The lumen is marked by an O. This plaque is causing high-grade stenosis, and the lumen is very small. The plaque has a large lipid core devoid of collagen.

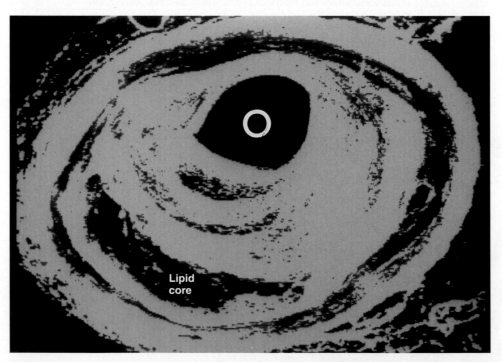

Figure 4-17. Collagen and Lipid in Plaques. There is high-grade stenosis and the plaque is very rich in collagen. There is a small lipid core deep in the plaque.

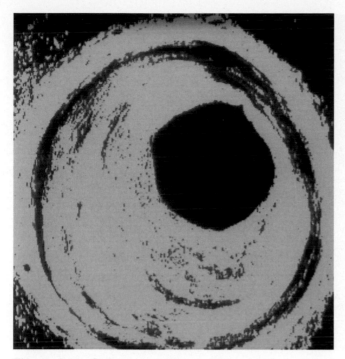

Figure 4-18. Collagenous Plaque. This plaque is almost entirely made up of collagen and does not have a lipid core.

proportion of all the plaques that have characteristics that endow a risk of thrombosis, i.e., a large core, is unique, although there is now data showing that having a high proportion of such vulnerable plaques is linked with being male, having high total serum cholesterol levels, and a low high-density lipoprotein (HDL) level (14). In any large group of individuals with stable exertional angina, there will be a subgroup of individuals in whom the vulnerability index, i.e., ratio of lipid-rich inflammatory plaques to fibrous plaques is high and a subgroup in whom the index is low and the majority of the plaques fibrous. The former will have a higher risk of a future acute ischemic event. The majority of individuals will lie between these extremes.

Some coronary stenoses are more complex but still result from atherogenesis alone. In such instances there may be more than one plaque with either completely separate lesions on opposite sides of the vessel or plaques that are superimposed on or overlap each other (Fig. 4-19).

In the majority of subjects with a history of stable angina in life, at necropsy there are arterial segments with the morphological hallmarks of having had a previous occlusive thrombus that has undergone organization and recanalization to leave several smaller lumens within the original vessel (15) (Figs. 4-20–4-22). These recanalized segments may or may not be related to the scars of previous myocardial infarction. In a pathology study of 54 cases with stable angina in life, 43 individuals had at least one such multichanneled lumen segments of artery; 33 of these segments were related to a myocardial scar, but 10 were not, indicating that occlusive thrombosis does not necessarily lead to infarction (13). In a similar manner, many subjects with stable angina have chronic subtotal or total occlusions (Figs. 4-23–4-27), often with local anastomotic flow in the adventitial vessels (16–18).

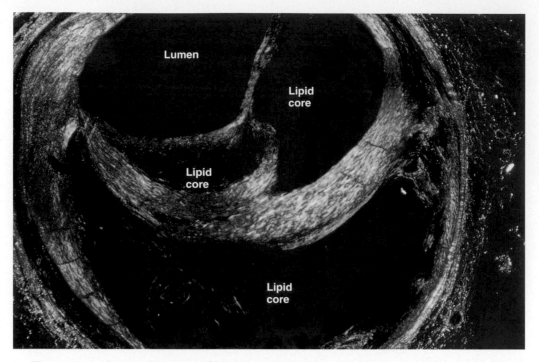

Figure 4-19. Plaque Superimposition. The collagenous structure of an arterial lesion is shown by Sirius Red viewed under polarized light. The lumen is top left. There are three separate lipid cores suggesting a plaque has formed over an existing plaque.

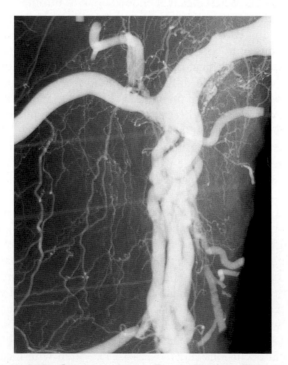

Figure 4-20. Coronary Artery Recanalization. The angiogram shows an abrupt transition from a relatively normal segment of artery to several channels closely related to and twisting around each other.

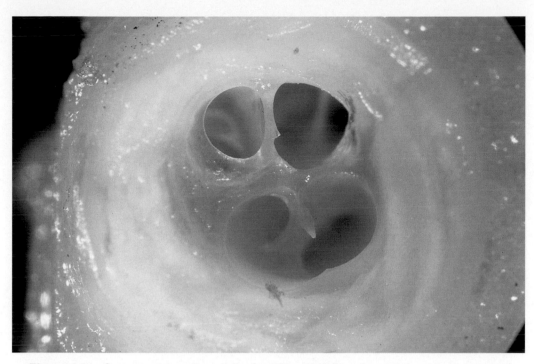

Figure 4-21. Coronary Artery Recanalization. The arterial lumen contains a honeycomb of new vascular spaces created by fibrous strands resulting from the organization of a previous occluding thrombus.

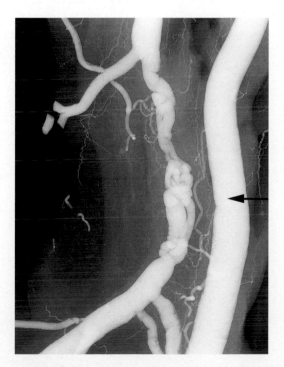

Figure 4-22. Coronary Artery Recanalization. The native coronary artery in the angiogram shows an irregular outline and, in a high-definition necropsy angiogram, it is possible to see it is due to a number of lumens spiraling around each other. *In vivo* angiography is far less able to identify the nature of these lesions—the lesion was bypassed and the smooth outline of the vein graft (*arrow*) alongside the native artery is seen.

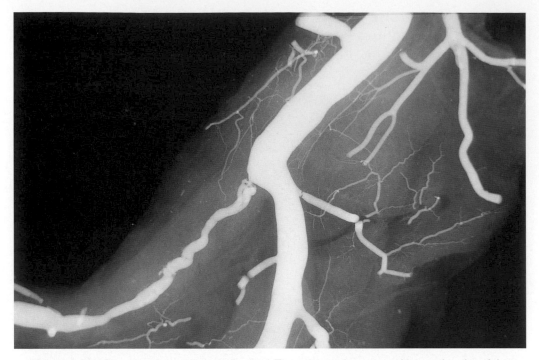

Figure 4-23. Coronary Artery Recanalization. There is an abrupt transition at the site of the origin of a major branch from a smooth-edged normal artery to a very fine tortuous lumen. This represents a previous occluding thrombus in which only a tiny single lumen was created in the recanalization process.

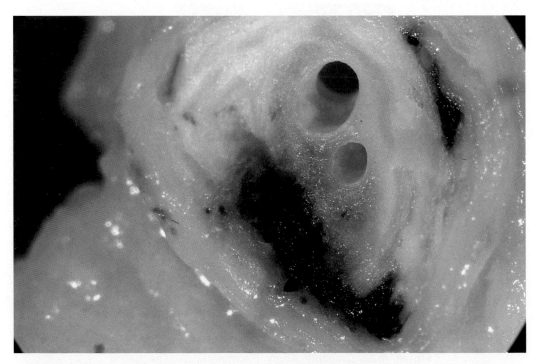

Figure 4-24. High-Grade Coronary Stenosis. Angiographic lesions such as those in Fig. 4-23 usually result from the healing of an episode of plaque thrombosis. In this lesion, the lumen is just a pinpoint in size within a mass of gray connective tissue within the original lumen. Deep within the plaque there is still residual thrombus enclosed by fibrous tissue.

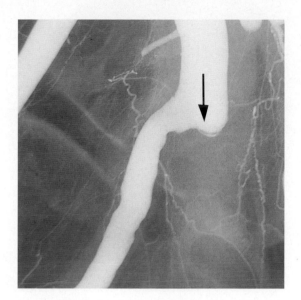

Figure 4-25. Chronic Total Occlusion. The angiogram shows a total occlusion (*arrow*) of the left anterior descending artery just distal to a patent major branch. The occlusion shows a smooth proximal edge and there is no evidence of filling in the more distal portion of the aorta.

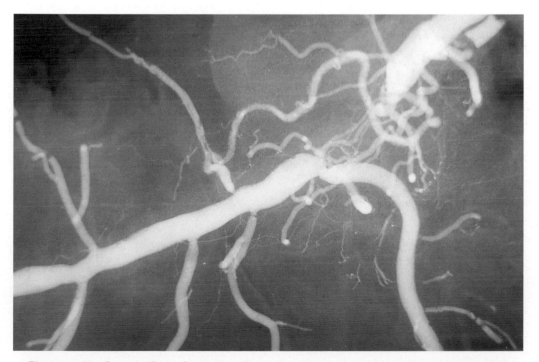

Figure 4-26. Chronic Total Occlusion. There is a short occluded segment of artery but there is good distal filling of an apparently normal artery by collaterals that have developed in the immediate area. Many of these local collaterals are in vessels within the adventitia.

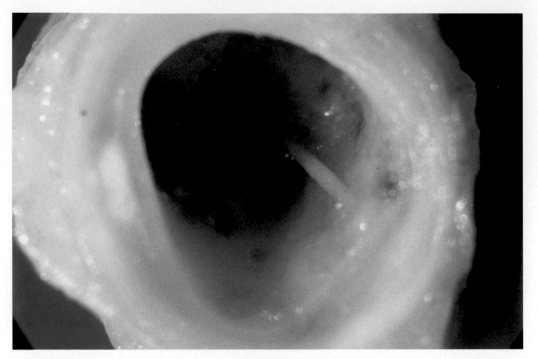

Figure 4-27. Chronic Total Occlusion. The artery is abruptly occluded by a smooth mass of fibrous tissue. Just visible within the mass is a strand of white tissue, which is a residue of the torn cap, indicating there had been plaque disruption in the past.

MECHANISMS OF PRODUCTION OF CHRONIC STENOSIS: COMPENSATORY DILATATION

Chronic stenosis is produced by a range of mechanisms. The simplest is that a plaque simply slowly increases in volume (Fig. 4-28) by the accumulation of lipid and the production of collagen to the point at which the capacity of the vessel wall to undergo compensatory dilatation (19,20) is exceeded. Intravascular ultrasound provides a means of studying compensatory dilatation *in vivo* and a number of aspects of the process are now clear (21–23). The effective upper limit of compensatory dilatation (vessel wall remodeling) is an increase of approximately 40% in the total cross-sectional area of the artery. A proportion of chronic high-grade stenoses do show this degree of increase in total cross-sectional area of the artery. Many stenoses, however, show a degree of compensatory dilatation (remodeling) that falls far short of these maximal values, and stenosis can be regarded as due, in part, to inadequate compensation. Adequate and inadequate compensatory dilatation occur in the same artery, suggesting that local plaque factors are responsible for the variation (24) (Fig. 4-29). One potential factor is adventitial fibrosis, which would limit vessel expansion. The heavy adventitial inflammatory infiltrate that develops behind some plaques may be a factor in increasing adventitial fibrosis. It is also suggested that paradoxical shrinkage of the artery at a site of stenosis (negative remodeling) to below the cross-sectional area of the normal artery is an important factor, particularly in the femoral artery (23). Personal experience suggests that this is rare in coronary lesions unless there is a virtually total chronic occlusion. In such segments, the internal elastic lamina has reverted to a wavy outline despite pressure fixation of the artery. It is, therefore, very difficult to exclude that the reduction in cross-sectional area of the artery is not an entirely secondary response to no flow rather than a primary event causing stenosis. In postangioplasty stenosis, a reduction of cross-sectional area of the vessel wall is more firmly established as a causative event (see p. 140). A second factor causing stenosis

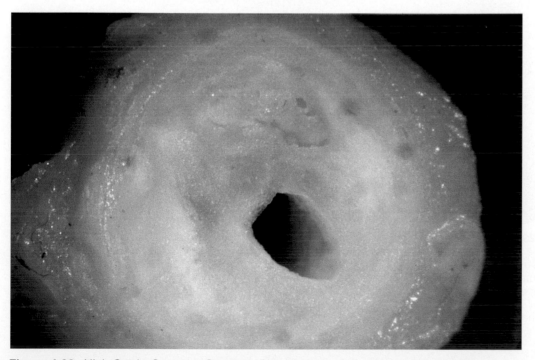

Figure 4-28. High-Grade Coronary Stenosis. The lumen is very small due to concentric intimal disease. In one segment of the thickened intima, lipid is deposited. The cross-sectional area of the artery overall was increased by over 30%, indicating compensatory dilatation had occurred and that stenosis was produced by a further increase in plaque size.

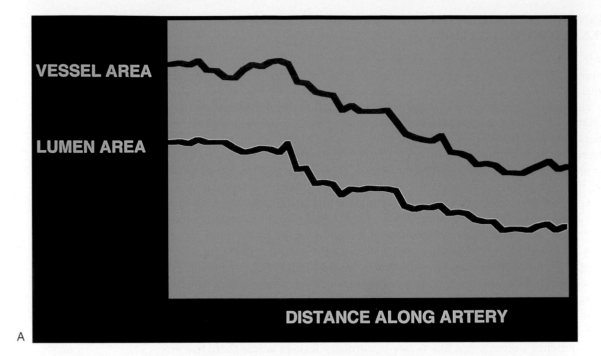

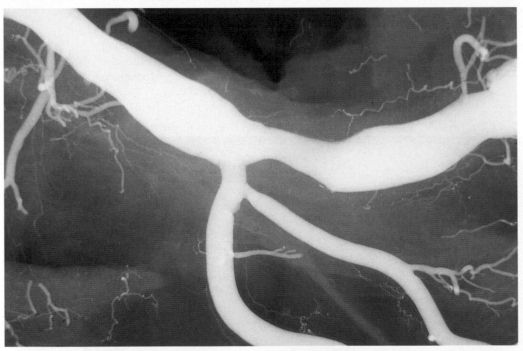

Figure 4-29. Compensatory Dilatation. **A.** In normal coronary arteries, the cross-sectional area of the vessel within the external elastic lamina and the cross-sectional area of the lumen run in parallel with a distal taper. The distance between the two curves is a measure of the intimal and medial volume. Perfuse fixed arteries distended at 100 mm Hg are an ideal method of studying compensatory dilatation. **B.** A postmortem right coronary angiogram showing from proximal to distal a normal artery segment, ectasia, normal artery, ectasia, and then a 50% diameter stenosis just distal to a side branch.

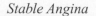

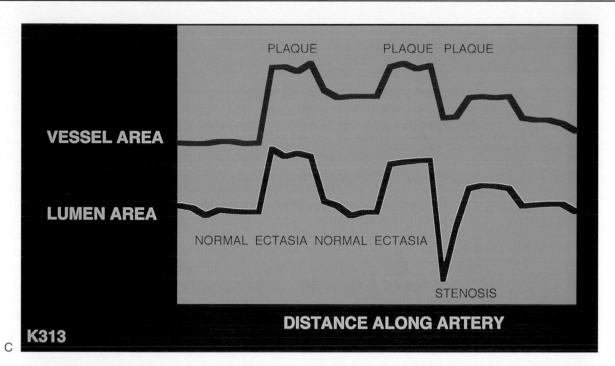

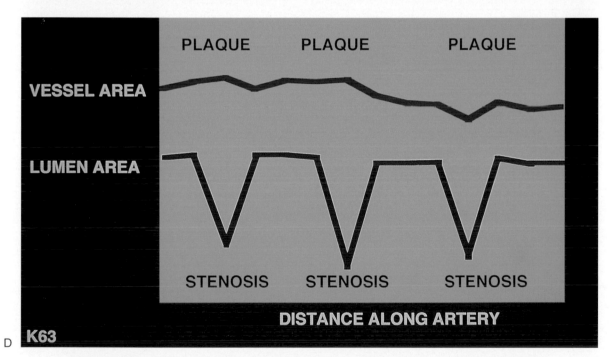

Figure 4-29. *(Continued).* **C.** Plot of lumen area against vessel cross-sectional area of the artery shown in (**B**). In the first two plaques the increase in vessel cross-sectional area (compensatory dilatation) has led to an increase in lumen size (mild ectasia). In the third plaque, although some compensatory dilatation of the artery had occurred, it was far less than for the first two plaques and failed to prevent stenosis. **D.** Plot of lumen area against vessel cross-sectional area in a right coronary artery with three discrete plaques all causing stenosis. No compensatory dilatation of any significant degree occurred in this artery.

is the rate at which plaque volume increases; if this rate exceeds the rate of remodeling of the arterial wall, stenosis will occur.

One factor producing rapid plaque growth is an episode of thrombosis that will stimulate rapid production of collagen and proliferation of smooth muscle cells. Many episodes of plaque thrombosis, whether this is by endothelial erosion or by disruption, are clinically silent but will lead to such rapid increase in plaque volume. The healed phase of an episode of previous thrombosis and disruption can be recognized by a number of pathological and histological features (Fig. 4-30). The dye Sirius Red binds specifically to collagen. Under polarized light, more recently formed collagen appears as a fine loosely arranged network of green-stained fibrils. Such areas are rich in smooth muscle cells arranged in a storiform pattern. More densely packed older type III-rich collagen appears yellow or white under polarized light. Image analysis of cross sections of plaques allows recently repaired breaks in the plaque cap to be recognized. The rapid expansion of a plaque that occurs in a postdisruption state may outstrip the speed at which the media can be remodeled, compensatory dilatation does not have time to develop, and stenosis occurs. One autopsy study of high-grade coronary stenosis unrelated to myocardial scars show 70% of the lesions to have evidence of a prior healed disruption. Taken overall, the mean amount of fibrous tissue in stenotic plaques is far higher than in nonstenotic plaques in the same individual (25,26). This has been used to suggest that fibrosis is the dominant mechanism in producing stenosis. It is, but in many cases has been triggered by prior subclinical episodes of thrombosis.

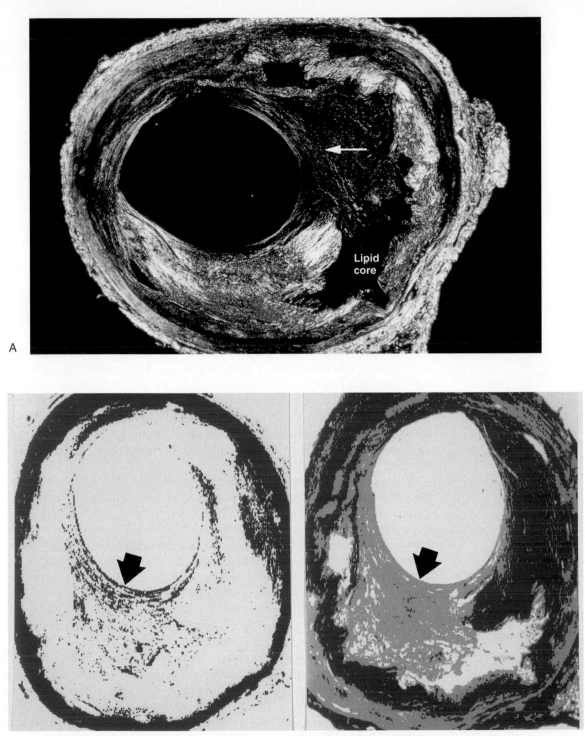

Figure 4-30. Healed Plaque Disruption. **A.** In this plaque stained by Sirius Red and viewed under polarized light, older collagen is yellow/white. A lipid core is present. The cap has a large defect that is filled by a more loosely arranged network of fine-green staining colla-gen (*arrow*). This represents the healing phase of a prior disruption. In (**B**), stained by immunohistochemistry for smooth muscle actin **(left)**, the media is red due to its high con-tent of smooth muscle cells. The area of new green collagen (*arrow*) is also rich in smooth muscle cells. Image analysis of the collagen from the Sirius Red stain **(right)** enhances the contrast between the magenta older and the green newer collagen.

VARIATIONS OF CORONARY ATHEROSCLEROSIS

A number of arterial diseases have affinities with atherosclerosis in that they share common cellular processes and are accentuated, although not necessarily initiated, by hyperlipidemia.

Ostial and Main Stem Coronary Stenosis

Ostial stenosis (27) appears to be a variation in coronary atherosclerosis in which intimal proliferation associated with foam cell infiltration on fibrosis develops predominantly at the junction of the coronary artery and aortic wall (Fig. 4-31). It is rare but appears to be more common in women than men. Pathological series in the past have tended to overreport the condition (28) due to visual and subjective opinions on a reduction in size of one orifice relative to the other. Main stem coronary disease has identical features to atherosclerosis in the other epicardial coronary arteries.

Coronary Artery Bypass Graft Disease

Saphenous vein grafts may undergo thrombosis within a very short period (less than 5 days) of insertion, usually as a result of low flow from the graft into the distal coronary artery (Fig. 4-32). In veins that remain patent and if good flow is established for more than a few days, there is the formation of a new intimal layer containing smooth muscle cells and fine elastin fibrils (Fig. 4-33). The endothelial surface is reconstituted after the extensive focal denudation of the endothelium that occurs during the operative procedure. The formation of this new intimal layer, which is not atherosclerosis per se, reflects both the adaptation of the vein to altered flow and pressure and the endothelial damage at surgery. Attempts to minimize the operative trauma to the graft during dissection in the leg, however, do not appear to significantly alter the adaptive response.

Vein grafts in which significant flow is established have a large lumen and a neointima that is easily recognized as a fibrous layer containing smooth muscle cells internal to the original wall of the vein. The media of the vein often undergoes considerable damage at the time of operation and may be largely replaced by fibrous tissue. Fibrosis and a giant cell granulomatous response to ligatures at the points where small side branches were tied off during the surgical removal may cause very localized strictures in the graft. It is doubtful whether the neointima formation in vein grafts is the cause of graft occlusion. Grafts are encountered at periods of a year after insertion in which the lumen is small and the whole graft small. Intimal thickening is present but it is likely that the major cause of occlusion is falling blood flow through the graft due to native vessel disease at the anastomoses.

The major cause of graft loss at periods after a year is atherosclerosis (29–31). With the passage of time, lipid-filled foam cells begin to appear in the most superficial (subendothelial) layer of the new intima (Fig. 4-34) and often involve virtually the whole of the graft inner surface. Endothelial loss develops with platelet deposition, and foam cell death occurs, releasing cholesterol into the tissues. Finally the graft is occluded by a pultaceous mass of thrombus admixed with cholesterol (Figs. 4-35, 4-36). The salient feature is the diffuse and friable nature of the intimal process. Localized plaque formation is unusual, although discrete stenosis sometimes appears at the anatomic sites with the native artery. Once atherosclerosis has developed, vein grafts appear to have very little capacity to undergo compensatory dilatation (22). Handling atheromatous grafts at redo surgical operations will release emboli of cholesterol crystals and thrombotic material (Fig. 4-37) into the distal vascular bed leading to focal myocardial necrosis and even regional infarction.

Internal mammary artery grafts undergo extensive remodeling over the first few weeks after insertion, increasing their external diameter to accommodate more blood flow. These arteries seem resistant to any atherogenic process and the stenoses, which

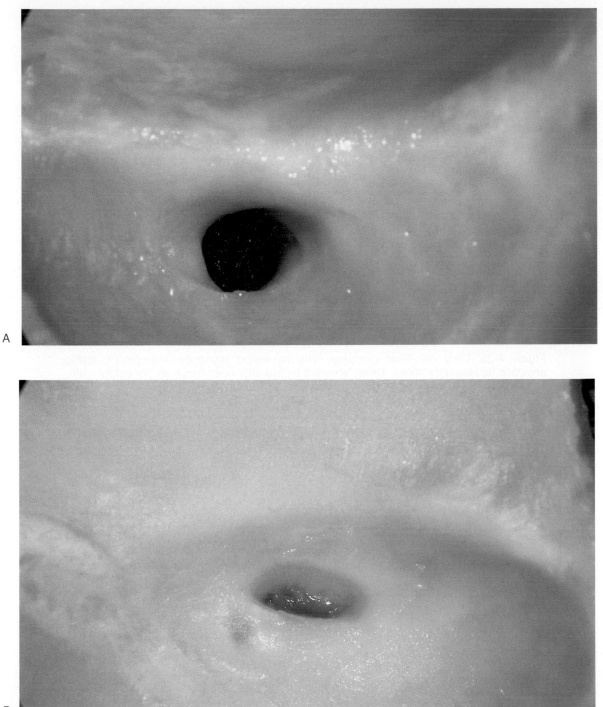

Figure 4-31. Ostial Stenosis. The right coronary orifice (**A**) is normal in size and shape, being widely patent. The left coronary orifice (**B**) is obliterated by white fibrous tissue.

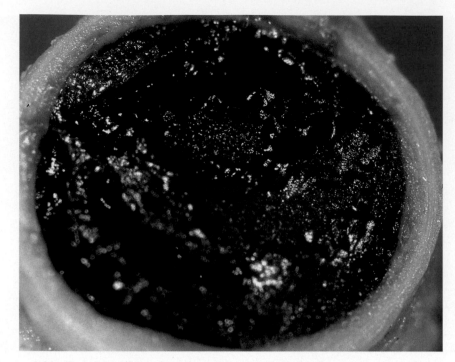

Figure 4-32. Early Vein Graft Occlusion. The thin-walled saphenous vein graft is totally occluded by recent thrombus. Death occurred 5 days after operation from low output state.

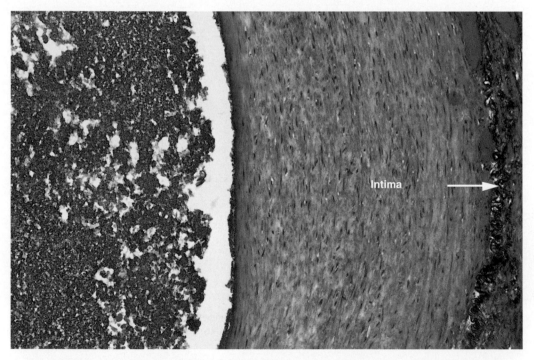

Figure 4-33. Neointima Formation in Vein Graft. In this histological section elastin has been stained black. The original medial intimal boundary in the wall of the graft is marked by an elastic lamina (*arrow*). The intima is at least twice the thickness of old vein wall and consists of smooth muscle cells embedded in collagen. The lumen, far left, contains gray postmortem angiographic medium.

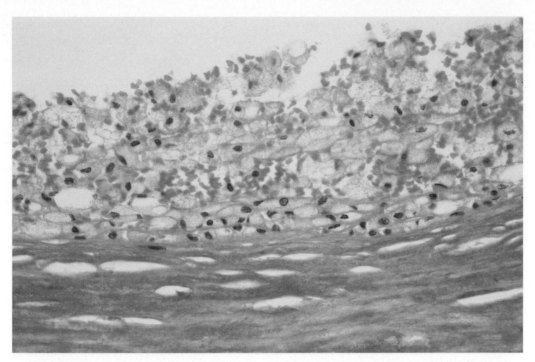

Figure 4-34. Vein Graft Atherosclerosis. The luminal aspect of the new intima is covered by a diffuse layer of macrophage foam cells, among which are entrapped red cells. The endothelial surface has vanished (hematoxylin and eosin).

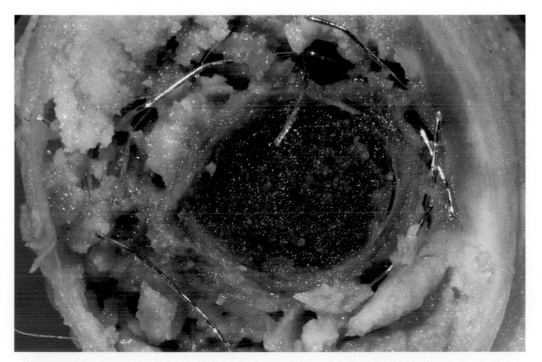

Figure 4-35. Vein Graft Atherosclerosis. A stent had been inserted for vein graft atherosclerosis. The figure shows the concentric thick layer of lipid-rich material into which the stent had been inserted. Thrombotic occlusion developed after a few weeks.

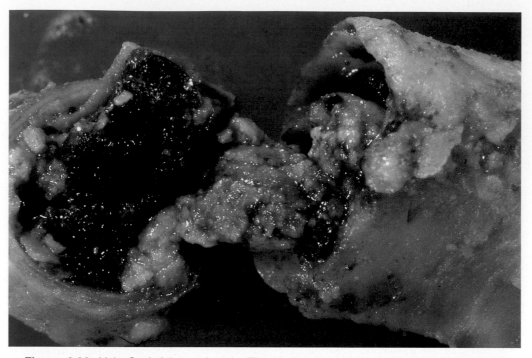

Figure 4-36. Vein Graft Atherosclerosis. The graft is occluded by a pultaceous mass of lipid admixed with thrombus. The material is very friable and can be very easily expressed from the graft by gentle pressure.

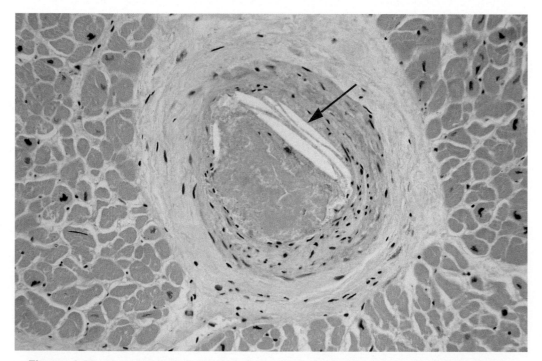

Figure 4-37. Myocardial Emboli after Redo Vein Graft. The intramyocardial artery is occluded by a mass of thrombus within which the elongated boat-shaped spaces (*arrow*) show that crystalline cholesterol was present in the embolus.

do rarely develop, are at the sites of anastomoses with the native arteries that have developed more atherosclerosis.

Familial Hypercholesterolemia

Genetic defects in the low-density lipoprotein (LDL) receptor of hepatocytes leads to the elevation of plasma cholesterol levels, which is typical of familial human hypercholesterolemia. The Watanabe rabbit is a genetic animal model of the same process. In both the rabbit and human disease, extensive atherosclerosis is produced (32) in which there is very diffuse intimal thickening associated with foam cell infiltration (see Fig. 3–18). Localized plaque formation is far less of a feature than in conventional atherosclerosis. The diffuse nature of the intimal disease leads to marked ectasia of the artery, often interposed with stenosis. Thrombosis is caused via the process of endothelial erosion rather than plaque disruption. Extension of the disease into small intramyocardial arteries is common. The foam cell infiltration also occurs in the aortic sinuses and at the supra aortic ridge where calcification will lead to aortic valve stenosis. Other causes of severe hypercholesterolemia, such as longstanding hypothyroidism and diabetes, can also lead to a similar rather diffuse form of atherosclerosis.

NONLIPID-CONTAINING ATHEROSCLEROSIS

Rare cases are encountered in which there is diffuse or focal coronary artery narrowing due to smooth muscle proliferation within the intima in the absence of any lipid or macrophages (14,33). The smooth muscle cells are characteristically arranged in a storiform pattern and there are large amounts of connective tissue mucins and proteoglycans present. The disease appears to be more common in younger females and has been described as a cause of sudden cardiac death. It is also responsible, when complicated by thrombosis, for isolated occlusions of the proximal left anterior descending artery in young females without the traditional risk factors for atheroma (Fig. 4-38). In some cases, the lesions appear rather focal but in others are associated with evidence of widespread recanalization, suggesting diffuse thrombosis had occurred (Fig. 4-39). Smoking has been implicated as one pathogenic factor and cases with more diffuse thrombosis are likely to be due to antiphospholipid antibodies (34).

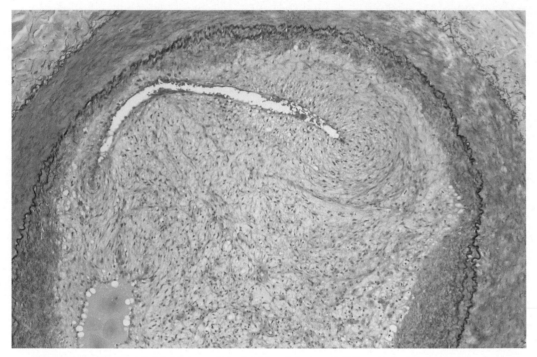

Figure 4-38. Nonlipid Atherosclerosis. The lumen of left anterior descending coronary artery is reduced to a slit by proliferating smooth muscle cells in the intima. No lipid or macrophages were present. Female aged 27 years with extensive anteroseptal scarring and cardiac failure needing transplantation.

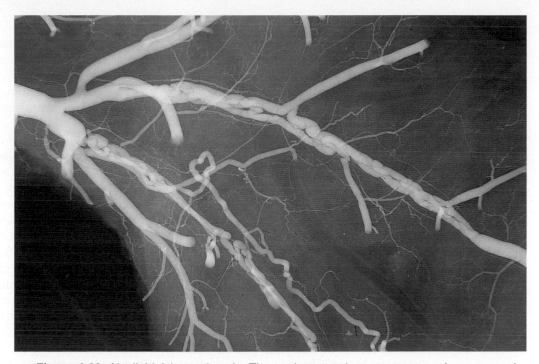

Figure 4-39. Nonlipid Atherosclerosis. The angiogram taken at necropsy shows several branches of the left anterior descending to have a multichanneled appearance suggestive of recanalization of thrombus. No lipid deposition was present histologically and the intimal proliferation was predominantly smooth muscle in type.

GRAFT VASCULAR DISEASE

Human cardiac allografts develop a form of coronary artery disease that has become the major cause of late deaths (35–38). The arterial lesions have many pathological processes in common with native vessel atherosclerosis, but the actual topography and morphology is very characteristic and different. The condition has a number of names, including graft vascular disease (GVD) and transplant-accelerated arterial disease (TACAD).

In its typical form, GVD is a diffuse concentric intimal thickening, which, over a period of years, steadily reduces the lumen size of the smaller epicardial arteries (Fig. 4-40). The even nature of the narrowing makes the disease difficult to appreciate in angiograms unless quantitative measurements are made over a period of some years. The disease also has a predilection for the first generation of intramyocardial arteries in the order of external diameter of 500–1000 μm (Fig. 4-41). In cases where these arteries are maximally involved, the only angiographic signs are very slow run-off from the pericardial arteries. The disease essentially begins as an "intimitis" in which intima is infiltrated by cytotoxic T lymphocytes. A phase of progressive smooth muscle proliferation in the intima then follows to produce the concentric luminal narrowing. Macrophage infiltration does not appear to be a primary event, but in the later stages, lipid-filled macrophages accumulate in a characteristic circumferential zone between the media and the thick intima. Lipid accumulation is more pronounced in subjects with hyperlipidemia and, therefore, potentiates rather than initiates the process. In donor hearts in which plaques already existed there appears to be accelerated growth, and focal stenoses may appear in epicardial arteries. Endothelial damage is widespread, and in the late stages thrombosis may develop. The myocardial lesions produced by TACAD are widespread small focal areas of necrosis and fibrosis rather than distinct regional infarcts. The pattern of distribution of graft vascular disease compared with native atherosclerosis is of a diffuse narrowing involving small epicardial and intramyocardial arteries rather than proximal focal stenosis.

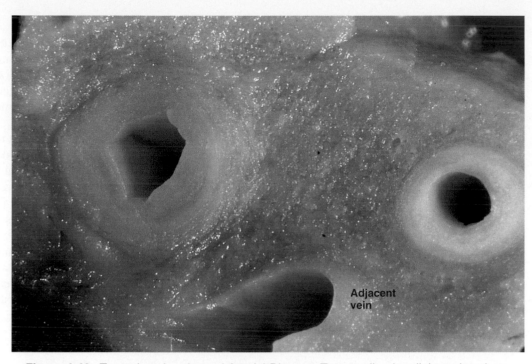

Figure 4-40. Transplant Accelerated Arterial Disease. Two small epicardial arteries show concentric wall thickening while an adjacent vein is thin-walled and normal. One of the arteries appears yellow due to deposition of lipid in the wall.

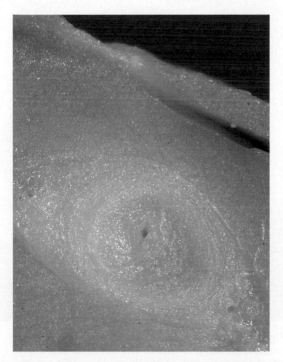

Figure 4-41. Transplant Accelerated Arterial Disease. A first generation intramyocardial artery with an external diameter of about 1 mm shows concentric wall thickening reducing the lumen to a very small aperture.

POSTANGIOPLASTY AND ATHERECTOMY RESTENOSIS

In balloon angioplasty there is virtually always tearing of the intima in or adjacent to the plaque (39). These intimal tears often extend into the media and may reach the adventitia. Intimal tearing is probably a prerequisite of successful angioplasty and is needed to enlarge the lumen (Fig. 4-42). In plaques that are eccentric, the segment of normal arterial wall is often stretched and thinned, providing another mechanism by which the lumen is increased in cross-sectional area.

The ubiquitous repair response (40–43) following mechanical trauma to the arterial intima is for smooth muscle cells to enter the proliferation cycle and undergo mitosis. Smooth muscle cells also migrate into the intima from the media, and this is enhanced if the media itself is torn. There is some evidence that the proliferative response in medial smooth muscle cells is greater and sustained for longer than that in the smooth muscle cells of the plaque itself. The proliferating smooth muscle cells are arranged in a storiform pattern initially embedded in a proteoglycan-rich matrix that is then replaced by collagen. The challenge for angioplasty has always been that a modicum of smooth muscle proliferation is needed for repair, but in at least 30% of cases the proliferative process and connective tissue synthesis continues to recreate a postangioplasty stenosis (Figs. 4-43, 4-44). Exactly the same repair process occurs after atherectomy. Medial damage also occurs in atherectomy and at least one third of samples removed contain at least one fragment of media.

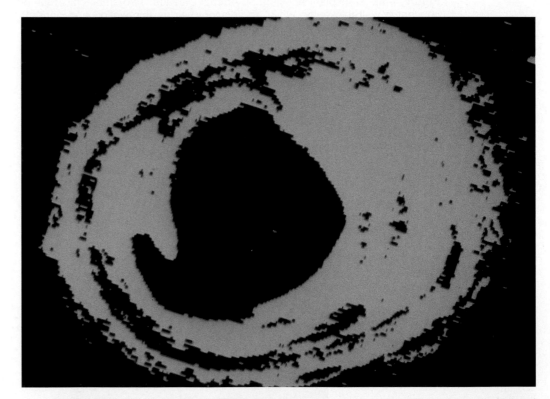

Figure 4-42. Postangioplasty State. In the coronary artery section the collagen is imaged to show collagen in yellow. The lumen is seen to be irregular in shape with an outpouching related to a smoothed-off intimal tear. The plaque structure is obliterated by fibrosis. Six months after angioplasty.

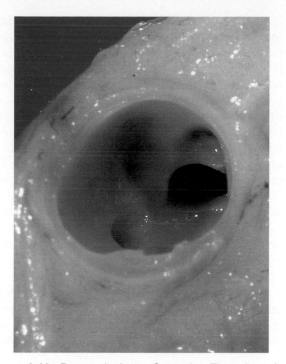

Figure 4-43. Postangioplasty Stenosis. The site of the angioplasty has been converted to a fibrous constriction in the vessel lumen.

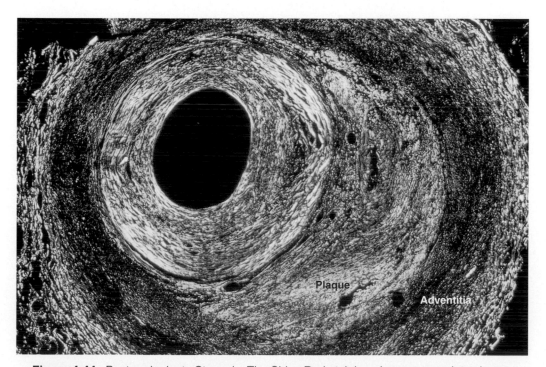

Figure 4-44. Postangioplasty Stenosis. The Sirius Red staining shows a complete circumferential zone of collagen surrounding the lumen as a fibrous cuff superimposed on the original plaque, which is replaced by fibrosis obliterating its architecture. The adventitia is also markedly thickened by fibrosis.

In cases in which a segment of normal arterial wall was stretched to enlarge the lumen, recoil over the next few days also contributes to restenosis. The adventitia is a remarkably strong structure with respect to tensile strength. In this regard it is salutory to remember that when endarterectomy is carried out the intima and the media is removed—the natural plane of cleavage in an artery is the medial adventitial junction not the intimal medial junction. In an artery after endarterectomy the wall is the adventitia until a neointima is created. The adventitia contains fibroblasts that can be invoked to produce more collagen after trauma. A further mechanism is described as responsible in part for postangioplasty stenosis. The ability of the vessel wall to undergo compensatory dilatation when a plaque develops within the intima has been previously discussed. After angioplasty, intravascular ultrasound suggests that the total cross-sectional area of the vessel may be substantially reduced by shrinkage. This negative remodeling will substantially reduce the amount of intimal smooth muscle proliferation needed to cause restenosis. The shrinkage is caused by fibrous tissue developing within the adventitia and media, presumably as a response to mechanical trauma. Retraction of scar tissue laid down in a repair process is well known in many other organs.

When stents are placed in an artery, smooth muscle proliferation creates a new intima that surrounds and incorporates the stent mesh to provide a smooth internal surface that ultimately reendothelializes. Stent stenosis is caused by proliferating smooth muscle cells extending into the lumen between the stent wires.

NONATHEROSCLEROTIC CORONARY ARTERY DISEASE

Coronary Artery Aneurysms

The definition of an aneurysm of the coronary artery varies. In the Coronary Artery Surgery Study (CASS) of over 20,000 subjects undergoing angiography, 4.9% were said to have coronary artery aneurysms (44). The definition used, however, was a diameter of one and one half times greater than a normal adjacent segment. Many would regard this definition as too broad, and includes what they would call ectasia due to atherosclerosis. Other definitions are more proscriptive and use the term *aneurysm* for a localized spherical or saccular dilatation up to three times greater than the normal adjacent artery. Such narrow definitions reduce the frequency to 0.2% of patients undergoing angiography (45). The great majority of diffuse and saccular aneurysms occur in the context of coronary arteries with evidence of diffuse atherosclerosis (Figs. 4-45, 4-46). Discrete aneurysms may follow procedures, such as atherectomy, where a portion of media has been removed (46). The pathogenesis of discrete aneurysms occurring in isolation in the absence of atherosclerosis is often impossible to determine in life or at autopsy. Single aneurysms are often regarded as congenital. An unknown proportion represent the final stage of a previous coronary arteritis, in particular, Kawasaki disease. The acute stage of the disease in childhood can easily be misdiagnosed in infancy as rubella, particularly in geographic areas where Kawasaki disease is rare. Late presentation of aneurysms (Fig. 4-47) in adults when thrombosis occurs is a well-recognized complication of Kawasaki disease in geographic populations where the disease is endemic in childhood (47). It is difficult to make clinical decisions on whether to surgically intervene in single aneurysms found on angiography. These localized aneurysms do thrombose and cause myocardial ischemia and infarction. The magnitude of the risk is impossible to predict because most are reported as single cases. Decisions have to be made based on whether myocardial ischemia can be shown and the area of myocardium at risk.

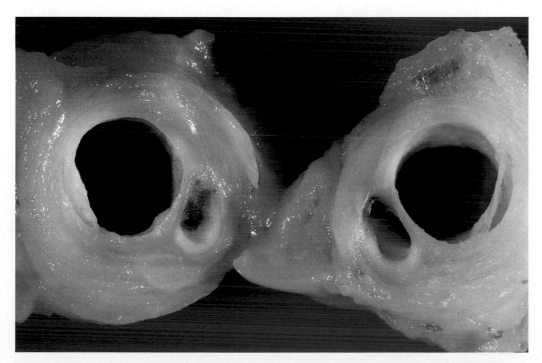

Figure 4-45. Coronary Artery Aneurysm. There is a small saccular aneurysm opening into the lumen by a narrow aperture. Such aneurysms are related to atherosclerosis and are a rare result of disruption of a plaque.

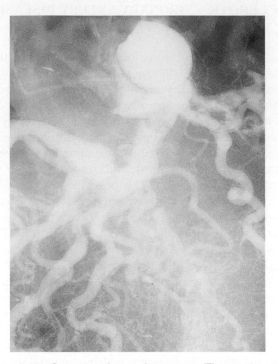

Figure 4-46. Coronary Artery Aneurysm. The postmortem angiogram from a man of 77 shows widespread ectasia with a localized saccular aneurysm. The age of the patient and the diffuse atherosclerosis associated with ectasia suggest the aneurysm is also due to atherosclerosis.

Isolated Coronary Artery Dissection

This entity is totally unrelated to aortic dissection and Marfan's syndrome (48). The condition is essentially the sudden development of a subadventitial hematoma (49) in a major coronary artery, which compresses the lumen from outside (Fig. 4-48). Many cases do not have an intimal tear, although such a tear is easily initiated, often by angiography in which the operator is horrified to see an artery dissect, despite perfectly easy cannulation and injection. Isolated coronary dissection presents either as sudden death or acute myocardial infarction in young individuals without risk factors for coronary atherosclerosis. Women are affected more commonly than men and a proportion of cases occur in pregnancy. The pathogenesis is totally unknown. Cases are described with a mild adventitial inflammatory infiltrate, but this is not a consistent finding. The disease does appear to have an acute phase in which the arteries are very vulnerable. For example, a patient with a spontaneous dissection of the left anterior artery may have the right coronary dissect at routine angiography. In subjects who survive, the arterial vulnerability wanes and the artery may return, angiographically, to normal. Such cases are one explanation for a myocardial infarct in which angiography a month later is normal.

Coronary Artery Bridging

In itself, bridging where a segment of a coronary artery is covered by a layer of myocardium before reemerging on the pericardial surface is a remarkably common finding at autopsy in hearts from subjects who have died of cardiac or noncardiac causes (50).

At least one third of "normal" hearts have at least one segment of bridging. The most common sites are the mid-left anterior descending and the left marginal coronary

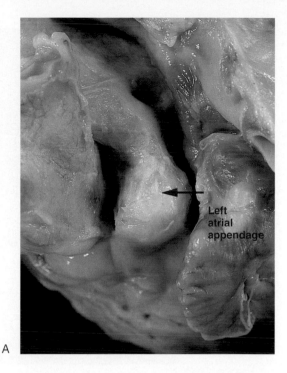

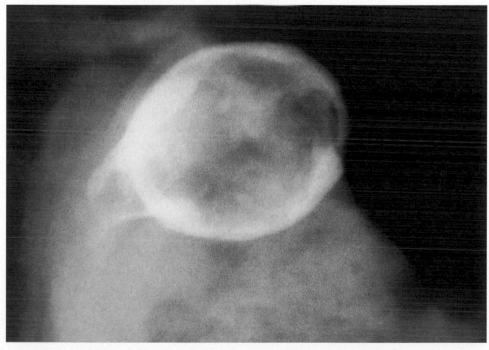

Figure 4-47. Isolated Coronary Artery Aneurysm. **A.** A localized saccular aneurysm (*arrow*) of the proximal left anterior descending coronary artery can be seen at the external surface of the heart between the aorta and the left atrial appendage. **B.** A plain x-ray shows the aneurysm to be calcified. The patient was aged 21 years and died suddenly. The fact that he came from a geographic area where Kawasaki disease is common makes this the likely diagnosis.

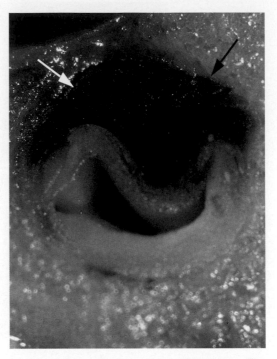

Figure 4-48. Isolated Coronary Artery Dissection. The proximal right coronary artery has a localized subadventitial hematoma (*arrow*) compressing the lumen. Sudden death.

artery. It is, therefore, clear that most bridged segments exert no abnormal affects and are asymptomatic. It is equally clear that a small proportion of myocardial bridges are not benign and are responsible for episodic ischemia or infarction. Many individual case reports (51–54) clearly show the bridging can produce abnormal flow. Symptomatic cases must have an additional factor responsible for a functional abnormality and one hypothesis is that the myocardium in the bridge is functionally abnormal, structurally abnormal, or abnormally innervated. An interesting facet of bridges is that the segment of artery in the tunnel is protected from atherosclerosis, but the immediately adjacent segments are more susceptible.

Anomalous Coronary Arteries

As described in Chapter 1, the normal state is for a coronary artery orifice to be present in the right and in the left aortic sinus. Some minor variations are without physiological significance. The left anterior descending coronary artery and the left circumflex coronary artery arising by two separate openings in the left coronary sinus is one example. A separate origin for the right ventricular conus artery in the right coronary sinus is another.

Other anomalies are more significant, but do not have pathophysiological significance, providing the artery that crosses from right to left, or vice versa, passes in front of the pulmonary trunk. Such anomalies have some disadvantages—the anomalous artery may be cut at surgery on the heart. If there is only a single coronary artery orifice a strategically placed plaque may jeopardize a very large area of myocardium. Nevertheless, these anomalies are usually associated with normal longevity.

A final group of anomalies (Fig. 4-49) are inherently dangerous (55,56). Any anomaly in which an artery crosses right to left or vice versa between the aorta and pulmonary trunk is at risk of intermittent ischemia and sudden death (Fig. 4-50). The segment of artery that crosses lies in a tunnel in the aortic media and may develop spasm as well as a slow intimal proliferation that finally occludes the artery. One coronary orifice in the aorta and another in the pulmonary trunk is also at risk (Fig. 4-51). An intramyocardial shunt develops and myocardial ischemia and fibrosis develop. Sudden death may occur in childhood but often there is good exercise tolerance up to sudden death as an adult. Individual case reports recording sudden death abound in the literature, leading to a view that when discovered at angiography these anomalies should be corrected in childhood. It has to be admitted, however, that some subjects with a coronary artery arising in the pulmonary trunk live into old age without correction.

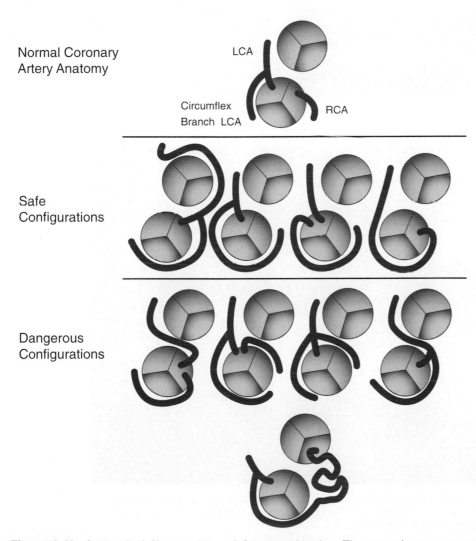

Figure 4-49. Anatomical Abnormalities of Coronary Arteries. The normal arrangement of the coronary arteries, safe and dangerous variants (RCA, right coronary artery; LCA, left coronary artery).

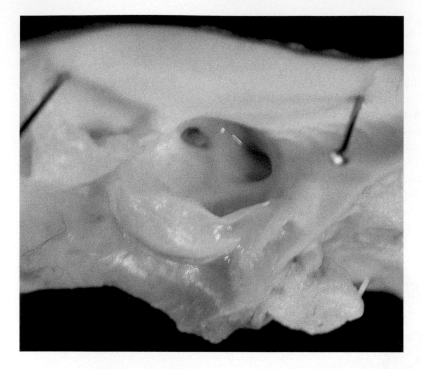

Figure 4-50. Abnormal Coronary Artery Orifices. Both coronary artery orifices are in one sinus. The right coronary artery crossed between the aorta and pulmonary trunk to reach its normal position. Sudden death after a history of occasional chest pain on emotion and exercise in a young subject.

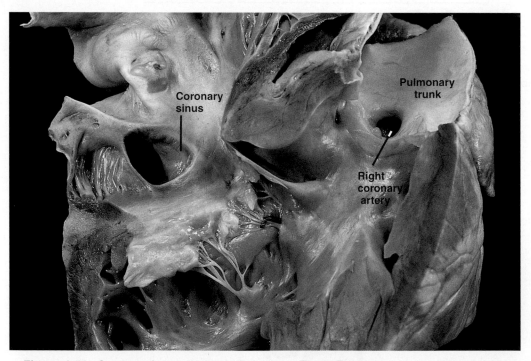

Figure 4-51. Coronary Artery Arising in Pulmonary Trunk. The right coronary artery arises from the pulmonary trunk. The coronary sinus is large. Sudden death on exercise—previously asymptomatic until death at age 37 years.

CORONARY ARTERY FISTULAE

Coronary artery fistulae may be acquired with shunts into the right ventricle after cardiac biopsy. Congenital fistulae (57,58) occur in any chamber or the coronary sinus (Fig. 4-52). The coronary artery tends to dilate and become tortuous with a very large lumen within which small mural thrombi often form.

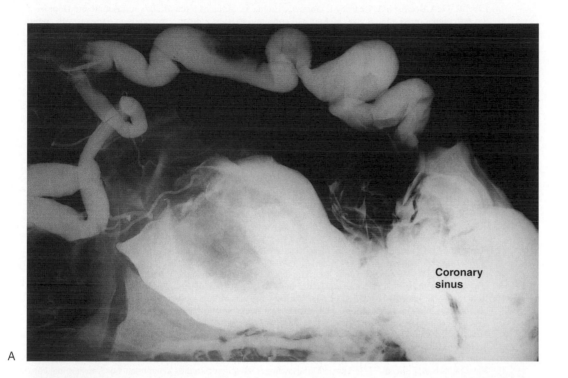

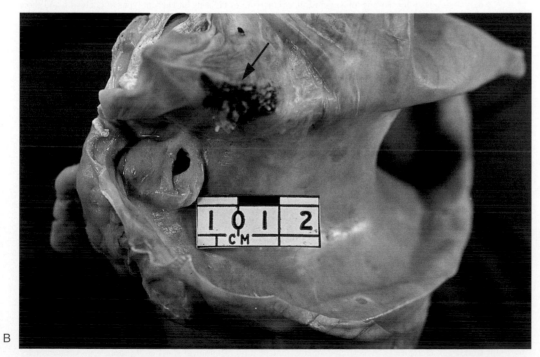

Figure 4-52. Coronary Artery Coronary Sinus Fistula. **A.** The left circumflex artery is dilated and tortuous and freely fills the coronary sinus at postmortem angiography. **B.** The coronary sinus has been opened from the posterior surface to show its large size and the dome-shaped papilla where the circumflex artery enters. There is mural thrombus (*arrow*) in the sinus.

REFERENCES

1. White C, Wright C, Doty D, et al. Does visual interpretation of the coronary angiogram predict the physiologic importance of a coronary stenosis. *N Engl J Med* 1984;310:819–824.
2. Ge J, Erbel R, Gerber T, Koch L, Haunde M. Intravascular ultrasound imaging in angiographically normal coronary arteries: a prospective study *in vivo. Br Heart J* 1994;71:572–578.
3. Alfonso F, Macaya C, Goicolea J, Iniquez A, Hernandez R, Zamorano J. Intravascular ultrasound imaging of angiographically normal coronary segments in patients with coronary artery disease. *Am Heart J* 1994; 127:536–544.
4. Erbel R, Ge J, Bockisch A, Kearney P, Gorge G, Haude M. Value of intracoronary ultrasound and Doppler in the differentiation of angiographically normal coronary arteries: a prospective study in patients with angina pectoris. *Eur Heart J* 1996;17:880–889.
5. Mann J, Davies M. Vulnerable plaque. Relation of characteristics to degree of stenosis in human coronary arteries. *Circulation* 1996;94:928–931.
6. Trask N, Califf R, Conley M, et al. Accuracy and interobserver variability of coronary cineangiography. A comparison with postmortem evaluation. *J Am Coll Cardiol* 1984;3:1145–1154.
7. Isner J, Kishel J, Kent K, Ronan JJ, Ross A, Roberts W. Accuracy of angiographic determination of left main coronary arterial narrowing. *Circulation* 1981;63:1056–1064.
8. Siegel R, Swan K, Edwalds G, Fishbein M. Limitations of postmortem assessment of human coronary artery size and luminal narrowing: differential effects of tissue fixation and processing on vessels with different degrees of atherosclerosis. *J Am Coll Cardiol* 1985;5:342–346.
9. Levin D, Gardiner G. Complex and simple coronary artery stenosis: a new way to interpret coronary angiograms based on morphologic features of lesions. *Radiology* 1987;164:675–680.
10. Kaski J, Tousoulis D, Haider A, Gavrielides S, Crea F, Maseri A. Reactivity of eccentric and concentric coronary stenoses in patients with chronic stable angina. *J Am Coll Cardiol* 1991;17:627–633.
11. Brown B, Bolson E, Dodge H. Dynamic mechanisms in human coronary stenosis. *Circulation* 1984;70: 917–922.
12. Saner H, Gobel F, Salomonowitz E, Erlien D, Edwards J. The disease free wall in coronary atherosclerosis: its relation to degree of obstruction. *J Am Coll Cardiol* 1985;6:1096–1099.
13. Hangartner J, Charleston A, Davies M, Thomas A. Morphological characteristics of clinically significant coronary artery stenosis in stable angina. *Br Heart J* 1986;56:501–508.
14. Burke A, Farb A, Malcom G, Liang Y-H, Smialek J, Virmani R. Coronary risk factors and plaque morphology in men with coronary disease who died suddenly. *N Engl J Med* 1997;336:1276–1282.
15. Roberts W, Virmani R. Formation of new coronary arteries within a previously obstructed epicardial coronary artery (intra-arterial arteries). A mechanism for occurrence of angiographically normal coronary arteries after healing of acute myocardial infarction. *Am J Cardiol* 1984;54:1361–1362.
16. Srivatsa S, Edwards W, Boos C, et al. Histologic correlates of angiographic chronic total coronary artery occlusions. Influences of occlusion duration on neovascular channel patterns and intimal plaque composition. *J Am Coll Cardiol* 1997;29:955–963.
17. Katsuragawa M, Fujiwara H, Miyamae M, Sasayama S. Histologic studies in percutaneous transluminal coronary angioplasty for chronic total occlusion: comparison of tapering and abrupt types of occlusion and short and long occluded segments. *J Am Coll Cardiol* 1993;21:604–611.
18. Kamat B, Galli S, Barger A, Lainey L, Silverman K. Neovascularization and coronary atherosclerotic plaque: cinematographic localization and quantitative histologic analysis. *Hum Pathol* 1987;18:1036–1042.
19. Glagov S, Weisenberd E, Zarins C, Stankunavicius R, Kolettis G. Compensatory enlargement of human atherosclerotic coronary arteries. *N Engl J Med* 1987;316:1371–1375.
20. Losordo D, Rosenfield K, Kaufman J, Pieczek A, Isner J. Focal compensatory enlargement of human arteries in response to progressive atherosclerosis. *in vivo* documentation using intravascular ultrasound. *Circulation* 1994;89:2570–2577.
21. Ge J, Erbel R, Zamorano J. Coronary artery remodelling in atheroslcerotic disease: an intravascular ultrasonic study *in vivo. Coron Artery Dis* 1993;147:151–266.
22. Nishioka T, Luo H, Eigler N, Berglund H, Kim C-J, Siegel R. Contribution of inadequate compensatory enlargement to development of human coronary artery stenosis: an *in vivo* intravascular ultrasound study. *J Am Coll Cardiol* 1996;27:1571–1576.
23. Pasterkamp G, Wensing P, Post M, Hillen B, Mali W, Borst C. Paradoxical arterial wall shrinkage may contribute to luminal narrowing of human atherosclerotic femoral arteries. *Circulation* 1995;91:1444–1449.
24. Mintz G, Kent K, Pichard A, Satler L, Popma J, Leon M. Contribution of inadequate arterial remodeling to the development of focal coronary artery stenoses. An intravascular ultrasound study. *Circulation* 1997;95: 1791–1798.
25. Roberts W. The coronary arteries and left ventricle in clinically isolated angina pectoris. *Circulation* 1976;54: 388–390.
26. Kragel A, Reddy S, Wittes J, Roberts W. Morphometric analysis of the composition of coronary arterial plaques in isolated unstable angina pectoris with pain at rest. *Am J Cardiol* 1990;66:562–567.
27. Stewart J, Ward D, Davies M, Pepper J. Isolated coronary ostial stenosis: observations on the pathology. *Eur Heart J* 1987;8:917–920.
28. Rissanen V. Occurrence of coronary ostial stenosis in necropsy series of myocardial infarction, sudden death and violent death. *Br Heart J* 1975;37:182–191.
29. Spray T, Roberts W. Changes in saphenous veins and as aorto-coronary bypass grafts. *Am Heart J* 1977;94: 500–516.
30. Bulkley B, Hutchins G. Accelerated atherosclerosis: a morphological study of 97 saphenous vein coronary artery bypass grafts. *Circulation* 1977;55:163–169.
31. Neitzel G, Barboriak J, Pintar K, Qureshi I, Clement J. Atherosclerosis in aortocoronary bypass grafts. Morphologic study and risk factor analysis 6 to 12 years after surgery. *Arteriosclerosis* 1986;6:594–600.

32. Roberts W, Ferrans V, Levy R, Fredrickson D. Cardiovascular pathology in hyperlipoproteinaemia: anatomic observations in 42 patients. *Am J Cardiol* 1973;31:557–570.

33. Farb A, Burke A, Tang A, et al. Coronary plaque erosion without rupture into a lipid core. A frequent cause of coronary thrombosis in sudden coronary death. *Circulation* 1996;93:1354–1363.

34. Ferro D, Pittoni V, Quintarelli C, et al. Coexistence of anti-phospholipid antibodies and endothelial perturbation in systemic lupus erythematosus patients with ongoing prothrombotic state. *Circulation* 1997;95: 1425–1432.

35. Johnson D, Alderman E, Schroeder J, et al. Transplant coronary artery disease: histopathologic correlations with angiographic morphology. *J Am Coll Cardiol* 1991;17:449–457.

36. Gao S, Alderman E, Schroeder J. Accelerated coronary vascular disease in the heart transplant patient: coronary arteriographic findings. *J Am Coll Cardiol* 1988;12:334–340.

37. Russell M, Fujita M, Masek M, Rowan R, Billingham M. Cardiac graft vascular disease: nonselective involvement of large and small vessels. *Transplantation* 1993;56:762–764.

38. Fujita M, Russell M, Masek M, Rowan R, Nagashima K, Billingham M. Graft vascular disease in the great vessels and vasa vasorum. *Hum Pathol* 1993;24:1067–1072.

39. Losordo D, Rosenfield K, Pieczek A, Baker K, Harding M, Isner J. How does angioplasty work? Serial analysis of human iliac arteries using intravascular ultrasound. *Circulation* 1992;86:1845–1858.

40. Casscells W, Engler D, Willerson J. Mechanisms of restenosis. *Texas Heart Inst* J 1994;21:68–77.

41. Simons M, Leclerc G, Safian R. Relation between activated smooth-muscle cells in coronary artery lesions and restenosis after atherectomy. *N Engl J Med* 1993;328:608– 613.

42. MacLeod D, Strauss B, de Jong M. Proliferation and extracellular matrix synthesis of smooth muscle cells cultured from human coronary atherosclerotic and restenotic lesions. *J Am Coll Cardiol* 1994;23:59–65.

43. Miller M, Kuntz R, Friedrich S. Frequency and consequences of intimal hyperplasia in specimens retrieved by directional atherectomy of native primary coronary artery stenoses and subsequent restenosis. *Am J Cardiol* 1993;71:652–658.

44. Swaye P, Fisher L, Llitwin P, Vignola P, Judkins M, Kemp H. Aneurysmal coronary artery disease. *Circulation* 1984;67:134–138.

45. Tunick P, Slater J, Kronzon I, Glassman E. Discrete atherosclerotic coronary artery aneurysm: a study of 20 patients. *J Am Coll Cardiol* 1990;15:279–282.

46. Desai P, Ro J, Pucillo A, Weiss M, Herman M. Left main coronary artery aneurysm following percutaneous transluminal angioplasty: a report of a case and a review of the literature. *Cathet Cardiovasc Diagn* 1992; 27:113–116.

47. Kato H, Inoue O, Kawasaki T, Fujiwara H, Watanabe T, Toshima H. Adult coronary artery disease probably due to childhood Kawasaki disease. *Lancet* 1992;340:1127–1129.

48. Davies M, Treasure T, Richardson P. The pathogenesis of spontaneous arterial dissection. *Heart* 1996;75: 434–435.

49. Basso C, Morgagni G, Thiene G. Spontaneous coronary artery dissection: a neglected cause of acute myocardial ischaemia and sudden death. *Heart* 1996;75:451–454.

50. Ishall T, Hosoda Y, Osaka T, et al. The significance of myocardial bridge upon atherosclerosis in the left anterior descending coronary artery. *J Pathol* 1986;148:279–292.

51. Felman A, Baughman K. Myocardial infarction association with a myocardial bridge. *Am Heart J* 1986;111: 784–788.

52. Tio R, van Gelder I, Boonstra P, Crijns H. Myocardial bridging in a survivor of sudden cardiac near–death: role of intracoronary doppler flow measurements and angiography during dobutamine stress in the clinical evaluation. *Heart* 1997;77:280–282.

53. Tauth J, Sullebarger T. Myocardial infarction associated with myocardial bridging: case history and review of the literature. *Cathet Cardiovasc Diagn* 1997;40:364–367.

54. Swartz E, Klues H, vom Dahl J, Klein I, Krebs W, Hanrath P. Functional characteristics of myocardial bridging: a combined angiographic and intracoronary Doppler flow study. *Eur Heart J* 1997;18:434–442.

55. Taylor A, Rogan K, Virmani R. Sudden cardiac death associated with isolated congenital coronary artery anomalies. *J Am Coll Cardiol* 1992;20:640–647.

56. Roberts W, Bethesda M. Major anomalies of coronary arterial origin seen in adulthood. *Am Heart J* 1986; 111:941–962.

57. Sunder K, Balakrishynan K, Tharakan J, et al. Coronary artery fistula in children and adults: a review of 25 cases with long-term observations. *Int J Cardiol* 1997;58:47–53.

58. Mavroudis C, Backer C, Rocchini A, Muster A, Gevitz M. Coronary artery fistulas in infants and children: a surgical review and discussion of coil embolization. *Ann Thorac Surg* 1997;63:1235–1242.

Subject Index

Subject Index

Page numbers followed by *f* refer to figures.